Recent Results in Cancer Research 50

Fortschritte der Krebsforschung
Progrès dans les recherches sur le cancer

Cancer Registry

Edited by

E. Grundmann and E. Pedersen

With 59 Figures

Springer-Verlag
Berlin · Heidelberg · New York 1975

Symposium of the "Gesellschaft zur Bekämpfung der Krebskrankheiten Nordrhein-Westfalen, e. V." Düsseldorf, April 6/7, 1973

Sponsored by the Swiss League against Cancer

ISBN 3-540-07008-7 Springer-Verlag Berlin · Heidelberg · New York
ISBN 0-387-07008-7 Springer-Verlag New York · Heidelberg · Berlin

Library of Congress Cataloging in Publication Data. Gesellschaft zur Bekämpfung der Krebskrankheiten Nordrhein-Westfalen. Cancer registry. (Recent results in cancer research; v. 50.) Proceedings of a symposium held in Düsseldorf, Apr. 6—7, 1973, and sponsored by the Swiss League against Cancer. Includes bibliographical references and index. 1. Cancer — Statistics — Congresses. 2. Diseases — Reportins — Congresses. I. Grundmann, Ekkehard, ed. II. Pedersen, Einar, 1917- ed. III. Schweizerische Nationalliga für Krebsbekämpfung und Krebsforschung. IV. Title. V. Series. [DNLM: 1. Neoplasms — Occurrence. 2. Registries. W1 RE106p v. 50 / QZ200 C216] RC261.R35 vol. 50 [RC262] 616.9'94'088s [616.9'94'071]. 74-23303.

Typesetting, printing and binding:
Konrad Triltsch, Graphischer Betrieb, 87 Würzburg, Germany.

Contents

Introduction

Planning and Evaluation of Oncologic Registries

Operation of Cancer Registries

Studies of Epidemiology

Closing Remarks

List of Participants

ANGLESIO, E., Registro dei Tumori per il Piemonte, I-10123 Torino, via Lagrange 2. Italy.

BARCLAY, T. H. C., Saskatchewan Cancer Commission, Allan Blair Memorial Clinic, 1555 Pasqua Street, Regina/Saskatchewan. Canada.

BARNES, A., National Vegetable Research Station, Wellisbourne/ Warwick, England.

BERNDT, H., Zentralinstitut für Krebsforschung, X 1115 Berlin-Buch, Lindenberger Weg 80, German Democr. Republic.

BJARNASON, O., University of Iceland, Dept. of Pathology. P. O. Box 150, Reykjavik/Iceland.

CLEMMESEN, J., Finseninstitutet/Cancerregisteret, Dk-2100 Copenhagen, Strandboulevarden 49, Denmark.

CORREA, P., Department of Pathology, LSU School of Medicine, 1542 Tulane Ave., New Orleans, La. 70112.

GRUNDMANN, E., Pathologisches Institut, D-44 Münster, Westring 17, Germany.

HAENSZEL, W., NIH, National Cancer Institute, Biometry Branch, Bethesda/Md. 20014, USA.

JUSSAWALLA, D. J., Indian Cancer Society, The Hon. Secretary, Tata Memorial Hospital, Parel, Bombay 12 DD, India.

KEDING, G., Gesundheitsbehörde, öffentl. Gesundheitsdienst 5, D-2000 Hamburg 13, Tesdorpfstr. 8, Germany.

LINDEN, G., California Tumor Registry, 2151 Berkeley Way, Berkeley/Ca. 94704, USA.

MARTINEZ, I., Department of Health, Cancer Control Program, San Juan/Puerto Rico, USA.

MUIR, C. S., WHO Internatl. Agency f. Research on Cancer, Div. Epidemiol. + Biostatistics. 150, Cours Albert Thomas, F-69008 Lyon, France.

NEUMANN, G., Landesverband Württemberg zur Erforschg. u. Bekämpfg. des Krebses e. V., D-7000 Stuttgart 1, Schickhardtstr. 35, Germany.

PEDERSEN, E., The Cancer Registry of Norway, Norwegian Radium Hospital, Oslo, Norway.

Ravnihar, B., Institute of Oncology, Ljubljana, Yugoslavia.

Saxén, E., III Department of Pathology, University of Helsinki, 00290 Helsinki 29, Finland.

Staszewski, J., Instytut Onkologii, Gliwice, Wybrzeźe Armii Czerwonei 15, Poland.

Tulinius, H., WHO, Internatl. Agency for Res. on Cancer, Unit Epidemiol. and Biostatistics, 150, Cours Albert Thomas, F-69006 Lyon, France.

Tuyns, A. J., WHO, same address.

Waterhouse, J. A., Birmingham Regional Cancer Registry, Queen Elizabeth Hospital. Birmingham B15 2TH, England.

Winkler, A., Medical Officer, WHO Cancer Unit, CH-1211 Geneva 27, Switzerland.

Introduction

The Pros and Cons of Cancer Registration

E. Grundmann

It may seem strange for somebody to hold a symposium on cancer registration and then submit a paper under the heading "The Pros and Cons of Cancer Registration." Indeed, this may be quite amazing to those of my colleagues who have been endeavoring for years or decades to provide a world-wide system of cancer registration. To be quite frank, this is exactly what I intended.

Generally speaking, as scientists we are convinced that the work we do is worth while. We are in fact supported in this attitude by public opinion, if one bears in mind that science is future-oriented. It may be said that science is a way for building the future, and that progressive-mindedness is - to use a modern word - "in." Nevertheless, we may somehow hesitate at this fashionable word. After all, science is not "in" in the way this word is interpreted by the younger generation. Indeed, this younger generation is much too sceptical whenever confronted with anything done by the older generation - and science is pursued primarily by the "establishment." Rather, it is "in" to criticize the system of society and, if possible, to overcome this system, which is responsible not only for many evils, but also for many illnesses.

However, in this paper I do not want to raise any doubts regarding the significance of cancer registration, but would prefer to encourage reflections on whether our trend towards cancer registration is really sensible. Science alone cannot be sensible. Anyone who succeeded in taking an optimistic view of the invention of dynamite and toxic gases was certainly convinced by Auschwitz or the atom bomb that the application of scientific knowledge can also have negative effects. There are now only a few places left on earth where people still tend to take a positive approach to these developments, and these areas are certainly not to be found in Europe, who bears many scars inflicted by science. That is why now, before doing any scientific work, we have to ask ourselves what the outcome of this work will be. This also applies to the registration of cancer.

The term "cancer registration" is made up of two words with an unpleasant meaning. In broad sectors of the population and among physicians in Germany, cancer is still regarded as an incurable illness causing either fear and unhappiness or resignation. So the best thing to do is not to use the word, not even when talking to a patient suffering from cancer.

Registration of human beings is also an unpleasant matter in our country. We had to be registered in various ways during the famous twelve years, which involved varying degrees of, but in many cases complete, loss of personal privacy. This is why most people in West Germany cannot be enthusiastic about anything like "cancer registry." They argue that any type of humanism, for which the well-being of mankind is the most important issue, is opposed to registration of any kind, particularly in the case of something as private as an illness. Incidentally, later in this paper I will refer to the fact that an illness is by no means a private affair. Our colleagues working in the public health service are well acquainted with the difficulties that arise both among the public and in parliament whenever the registration of diseases is debated. As, in our opinion, the state must serve the individual, and not vice versa, society must make due allowance for the interests of the individual; after all, no one would like to see his own name published in a list stating that he is a sick man, possibly even suffering from cancer.

Public opinion on scientists in general and on physicians in particular is much more sceptical in West Germany than, for example, in the Anglo-Saxon countries. Therefore, when colleagues who have come to this symposium from abroad ask why we have only two cancer registries in Germany, both situated in rather small areas (Hamburg and Saarland), this public scepticism is the only explanation we can give. By "the public" I mean not only the nonphysician, but also most of our colleagues. It might be of interest to doctors in Germany that at the beginning of this century the German Reich was the leading country in the field of cancer registration. On Sunday, February 18, 1900 at 12.15 p.m., eleven medical councillors met at the Ministry of Education in Berlin to found a "Comité für Krebsforschung" (Committee for Cancer Research). The following year, on November 14, 1901, Dr. Wutzdorff, head of department of the Kaiserliches Gesundheitsamt in Berlin, gave a report "Über die Verbreitung der Krebskrankheit im Deutschen Reich" (the Distribution of Cancer in the German Reich). In this report, details on the type of statistics to be used and on the first results obtained were specified, such as the increase in cancer mortality in Prussia between 1876 and 1898, which was roughly 120%, compared with a population increase of approximately 24%. At that time, people were most prone to cancer in the seventh decade of life. It is interesting to note that in 1892 there were more deaths due to malignant growth in certain states in Southern Germany and in Saxony than in the other states.

The first successful registration of cancer was published by Rigoni-Stern in 1844 in Verona, which at that time was part of the Austro-Hungarian Empire. Stern confined himself to the types of cancer that are externally visible, i.e. of the skin, the mamma, and the uterus. He also provided the first valid data as to the frequency of cancer at various ages, data which incidentally do not differ very much from the data available today. In 1840, it was reported for the first time by Rechnitz, of Pest, in the Austro-Hungarian Empire, that cancer of the lip was at that time the most common type; in 1850, Melzer reported on the frequency of this type of cancer among 28,800 hospital patients examined between 1787 and 1849. These results (1) were obtained thanks to the revolutionary hospital organization set up in those days in the Austro-Hungarian Empire by van Swieten on behalf of the Empress Maria Theresia.

Thus, history shows that cancer registration is by no means a "modern invention" but a real problem that has been confronting the world ever since modern therapeutic methods were first applied to people suffering from cancer. Nevertheless, it must be admitted that cancer registration is not necessarily supported by this historical development, considering that not everything done in the past is still expedient today. Before attempting to make some comments regarding the value of cancer registration, I should refer to the various types of cancer registries. There are basically three different types:

1) hospital registries,
2) central cancer registries, and
3) regional medical programs.

Hospital registries record all cases of cancer observed at a hospital. In a way, they act as a basis for the more comprehensive types of registries. To ensure that these registries can be evaluated with a reasonable degree of reliability, they must fulfill certain conditions, which are discussed in later papers. A central cancer registry is based on the co-operation of several hospitals in a certain area, the objective of such a registry being to record,compare, and evaluate all the data available. A regional medical program allows statistics on larger geographical areas and investigations on rare types of tumor.

Whereas the first type of registry, i.e. the clinic or hospital registry, provides a survey of the work done by an individual hospital, the conclusions that can be drawn on the basis of a central cancer registry have a far greater impact. In this paper, I would like to mention just four aspects of their value:

1) Regional comparison makes it possible to study the quality of diagnoses. This also applies to semimalignant tumors, which often confront pathologists with considerable difficulties when they attempt to specify their exact nature. Moreover, it must be considered in this context that the relevance of a diagnosis of the so-called carcinoma in situ is still unknown (4).

2) Comparison of various types of treatment makes it possible to determine statistically which therapy will be optimal for a given tumor patient. For example, the efficiency of a new chemotherapeutic method can be judged only with the aid of a comparison of this kind, so-called blind studies or even double blind studies also being required for tumor patients.

3) The exchange of results between the individual hospitals could encourage adoption of the best diagnostic and therapeutic methods.

4) Data compiled on age distribution, sex distribution, regional occurrence rates of certain types of tumors, etc. within large-scale statistical studies make it possible to get an idea of the epidemiology and thus, in some cases, of the etiology of malignant tumors. The epidemiological studies carried out in recent years (e.g. 3), would not have been possible without the help of cancer registries.

I believe that these four aspects - to which further ones could certainly be added with no difficulty - do not merely prove the value of cancer registries, but actually show that they are absolutely necessary. It must be borne in mind that every patient with cancer who lives in the area covered by such a registry will derive immediate benefit from cancer registration, since at least the first three aspects referred to above can have a direct effect on the treatment of a tumor patient. After all, every layman expects his doctor to use the best diagnostic and therapeutic methods to cure him of a disease, but doctors cannot know which diagnostic and therapeutic methods are best, if there is no opportunity for comparison.

Thus, cancer registration must be regarded as a means of improving the treatment of patients. Moreover, it provides the basis for studies on the etiology of cancer and on its pathogenesis, in this way helping us to find the path towards the prophylaxis of cancer. It must also be considered that if the results of cancer registration are made available to the public in a reliable and appropriate manner, they will serve the additional function of promoting public health education. In view of the scepticism prevailing in West Germany against intrusions upon the privacy of the individual, we must consider in what way we shall be able to attain a workable registration of cancer. There can be no doubt that the approaches taken so far in Hamburg and the Saarland must serve as the starting point. It should be mentioned in this context that Hamburg set up the world's first central cancer registry in 1927.

In my opinion, an approach we could adopt in West Germany is as follows: Every cancer patient has to attend a hospital sometime for the purpose of diagnosis or therapy, or at least his tumor is examined in a pathology laboratory. Accordingly, registration can be performed in the hospitals (hospital registries). At the hospital, a card is filled in for each cancer patient and is then filed. Professional secrecy can be guaranteed by using cards consisting of two parts: the first shows the full name and address of the patient, whereas the second part (or, for example, the copy) shows only the first letters or the initials, the date and place of birth, and the patient's number. With modern methods of data compilation, it is then possible to enter all the important details on the patient himself and his disease on the rest of the card. The first card with the patient's name and address is kept at the hospital, while the second one must be sent to the central or regional registry. There, the personal data of the patient are stored in an immediate-retrieval system, so that if a second report is submitted for the same patient, a different hospital (or a Pathology Institute) is able to determine whether the patient has already been entered in the registry or not. In this way it is possible to avoid any duplication of entries and also to ensure that the office where the patient's illness is evaluated receives all the data necessary for this purpose without being informed of the patient's identity.

I believe that we could apply the "triple approach", i.e. a method based on geographic, climatic and qualitative criteria, proceeding as follows:

> Certain selected clinics and hospitals should be given the opportunity of setting up local cancer registries, using uniform registration sheets to be prepared by an ad hoc committee along the lines of the system applied in Hamburg or the Saarland or in various foreign countries.Each West-German state should set up a so-called central cancer registry with the objective of providing advice for the individual hospital registries and of compiling and evaluating their data as far as possible.
>
> In order to clear the path for a scientific evaluation of the data compiled in all West-German states, the German Federal Republic as a whole should form one "registration area." In my opinion, the "Deutsches Krebsforschungszentrum" in Heidelberg would be the right organization to take over this task.

Three preliminary steps seem to be necessary before a program such as that described above can be realized:

1) The hospitals selected must be convinced that cancer registration is a worthwhile task, as this would create the right basis for cooperation;

2) Colleagues must be prepared for the task of cancer registration by special training courses, possibly held abroad;

3) Funds must be made available for cancer registration, whether by the governments, by the "Deutsche Forschungsgemeinschaft," or by other institutions that promote research.

It is high time that we in West Germany started the registration of cancer on a broad base. As I have already emphasized, cancer is by no means a solely private problem. To a very great extent it is a problem of significant socio-medical relevance. I would not like to go into the annual death rates due to malignant tumors in detail. Indeed, it is quite sufficient to emphasize that such malignant tumors take the second place in mortality statistics, exceeded in number only by circulatory diseases. Moreover, I have not attempted to present any data as to the enormous expenditure for the diagnosis and treatment of cancer. There can be no doubt that this expenditure is quite astronomic compared with the funds required for the setting up and maintenance of registration program. I am quite sure there are further questions concerning the pros and cons of cancer registration. But I am equally sure that the pros will increase and the cons will fade for every person who reads the papers in this volume.

References

1. CLEMMESEN, J.: Role of registries in cancer control. Historical perspectives. Oncology 5, 335 (1970).
2. Comités für Krebsforschung. Verhandlungen. Dtsch. med. Wschr. 27, 307 (1901).
3. GRUNDMANN, E., TULINIUS, H.,(Ed.): Current problems in the epidemiology of cancer and lymphomas. Rec. Res. Cancer Res. 39, 248 (1972).
4. HAMPERL, H.: Preinvasive carcinoma. Rec. Res. Cancer Res. 44, 53-56 (1974).
5. RIGONI-STERN, D.: Fatti statistici relaviti alle mallattie cancerose che servirono di base alle poche cose dette dal dott. Servire Progr. Pathol. Terap. Ser. 2. 2, 507 (1842).
6. WUTZDORFF: Über die Verbreitung der Krebskrankheit im Deutschen Reich. Dtsch. med. Wschr. 28, 161 (1902).

Unification of Hospital-Based Cancer Registries

A. Winkler

The present trend for collaboration work in cancer control activities on national and international levels between cancer institutes or cancer departments is obvious. The importance of such work is now well recognized, and many problems could not be solved without this collaboration. Even when such an actitivity is undertaken, however, as it has been by the Cancer Unit of WHO over the past few years, it quite soon becomes obvious that there are inherent differences between institutes, which make such an approach rather difficult, if not sometimes impossible. Examination of these differences exposes common roots. These common roots, which are the sources of difficulties in any attempt at international cancer control, lie principally in the absence of standardization - unification in the broadest sense, and include

- differences in pathological nomenclature used in cancer,
- different methods for the classification of cancer,
- different staging of cancer, and
- differences in the methods used for the assessment of data for evaluation and presentation of end results, etc.

It was felt, therefore, that if the Cancer Unit were to help in promoting the work of cancer control, it should attempt to draw up some guidelines, that would be acceptable to as many institutions and countries as possible, and that WHO was probably the most appropriate organization to do this. The program for unification of the pathological nomenclature is a current, large, and long-term project of the Cancer Unit, and the very clear-cut aim of this project seems to be acquiring more and more recognition. In our present exponentially developing world a common language is necessary for understanding, and whatever criticism there is of the "teething troubles" of these activities, I believe the final aim of a unified nomenclature will be reached.

We felt that a further step should be an attempt to standardize hospital cancer registries, which would naturally use all those elements for which unification or standardization is already achieved or recommended (ICD, MOTNAC, TNM, etc.).

It is well known that in some countries and some cancer institutions or larger hospitals, hospital-based cancer registries are already well established, are fully computerized, and are able to provide data for many types of studies. Most of these, however, have been created and established at the local cultural and educational level and for the local and national need and thus their stores of data cannot be simply transferred and utilized in other different geographic, ethnic or cultural situations without substantial changes.

There are several publications on hospital-based cancer registries and tumor registries, those published from 1955 onward (1-21) being particularly valuable. All these publications describe the usefulness of registries of this kind, enumerating the justifications for them and their aims[1], giving recommendations on how to establish them and estimates of the cost, etc. But nearly all of them are based on local standards and are tailored to the local level in each case.

With this in mind, the Cancer Unit decided to approach the problem in a rather different way. At the first discussion on this subject, held in November 1971 in Geneva, three main aspects were considered:

1) the registry should be applicable in any developed or developing country;
2) the type of registry finally proposed should be ready for immediate use; and
3) it should overcome language barriers.

In several institutions, registration is performed by paramedical personnel and particularly in developing countries, even the "know-how" is sometimes completely absent, even though the large cancer institutes concerned are fully equipped and functional. This statement is based on the study of 26 hospital cancer registries covering developed and developing countries in Europe and the Eastern Mediterranean Region of WHO.

There were three levels of technical sophistication:

1) simple cards kept in alphabetical order and cancer site order. This type of registration is used in 14/26 registries, 6 of which are in developed countries in Europe;
2) hand-sorted punched cards, used in 4/26 registries;
3) computer facilities, used in 8/26 registries.

The total number of different information items collected in these 26 registries was 97. The maximum number of information items collected in a single institute was 84 and minimum 5; the average number of items of information recorded in one institution was 35, with a rather wide variation. However, incredible as it seems, 2 registries contain no information at all on diagnosis. The ICD code for diagnosis is not used in 5 registries, one of which is in a highly developed country. Only 14 registries collect follow-up data. Only 11 registries offer direct data on survival; 16 registries indicate the date of death, but only 8 of them also include the cause of death. Two registries, in countries where it seems irrelevant, code the religion, and only one of the countries where the religion could be relevant with reference to circumcision and dietary habits gives the data on religion. In only 16/26 registries are the post-mortem findings notified. Some of the registries have a rather elaborate card on X-ray therapy, but the master card does not include the diagnosis. Three registries, which do not have any provision for histological diagnosis, record the blood groups.

The enumeration of inconsistencies, omissions, and differences in the data collected is by no means exhausted by these few examples. But even this short paragraph gives a picture of the present situation in hospital cancer registries. It is necessary to add, of course, that the definition of information collected varied and that the terminology and patterns of preprinted forms show such a wide diversity that comparison is very laborious and sometimes impossible. More details are given in Appendix II.

---

[1] see Appendix I

This study revealed that

1) the aim of hospital cancer registries is not well understood and
2) in many instances a registry is created without prior study or understanding of the subject;
3) the composition of data to be recorded, and particularly their definition and terminology, varies widely and
4) many of the data are meaningless.

In addition, many countries from which we obtained hospital registry forms do not have a population-based cancer registry, so that the hospital registry is the sole source of cancer data. Furthermore, there are many countries in which the identification of patients is extremely difficult, sometimes impossible, and special arrangements are necessary to allow identification. These countries often have specialized cancer institutes, however, some of which are well equipped. We believe, therefore, that a hospital cancer registry established in these institutes may very well serve as a nucleus and, later, as a source, for future population-based cancer registries.

During a second consultation on hospital-based cancer registries, the information to be coded was divided into two types:

1) core information (26 items) and
2) optional information (23 items).

The total number of items of information is thus 49. In collaboration with the WHO Data Processing Unit, the Cancer Unit is currently preparing a card suitable for use at two levels of sophistication:
a) manual use of punched cards - for those institutions which do not currently have any means of computerizing their data. Only 23 items of information can be coded on the cards in this system, and
b) computerization - the card is prepared in such a way that it can be read directly by a computer-card key punch operator.

If, for example, the hospital has no access to computer facilities, but wishes to retain the information recorded, it can code all the information and punch only the items for which hand-punching is available. At a later stage, when computer facilities are available to the institute, the transfer to this level of sophistication would be easily made and would not involve any loss of coded information or change in design. The language barrier can be overcome by allocation of a definite number to each item of information coded.

The practical value of this card will be tested in 15 cancer institutes over six months. It may prove to have many deficiencies and shortcomings, which will have to be discussed again with the users, WHO staff, and consultants before a final proposal can be made. There is reason to hope that this first step in standardization of hospital-based registries will have a favourable effect on the comparability of different data collected in cancer institutes or cancer departments of hospitals throughout the world.

References

1. BRANDON, G.: Cancer registry generalities. Acta Cancerol. (Lima). 7, 2, 82-89 (1968).
2. BRUMAGE, W. S.: The cancer registry - a vital hospital tool. Texas Med. 62, 8, 29-30 (1966).

3. COOK, G. B., WATSON, F. R.: The hospital-based tumor registry - a survey of operational characteristics. Bull. Amer. Coll. Surg. 55, 17-21 (1970).
4. EISENBERG, H.: The value of a central tumor registry. Ind. J. Cancer, 3, 2, 75-93 (1966).
5. FAULKNER, K. E., LEYLAND, L., WOFINDEN, R. C.: Cancer registration: a cross-check on completeness of cancer mortality information at South Western Regional Hospital Board Cancer Records Bureau. Medical Officer. 118, 12, 147-148 (1967).
6. FEINSTEIN, A. R., PRITCHETT, J. A., SCHIMPFF, C. R.: The epidemiology of cancer therapy. 4. The extraction of data from medical records. Arch. Int. Med. 123, 5, 571-590 (1969).
7. GRAHAM, T. O., AUSMAN, R. K.: A computer approach to cancer patients follow up. J. Surg. Oncol. 1, 1, 13-18 (1969).
8. HADDAW, A. J.: The coverage achieved by the cancer registration scheme in the Western Hospital Region of Scotland in 1965. Health Bull. (Edin.) 26, 2, 10-12 (1968).
9. HAENSZEL, W., HON, N. B.: Statistical approaches to the study of cancer with particular reference to case registers. J. of Chron. Dis. (St. Louis). 4, 6, 589-599 (1956).
10. HOIMAN, D. O.: The tumour clinic and the tumour clinic registry. J. Iowa State Med. Soc. 61, 94-97 (1971).
11. KOSTKA, Z.: Rozbor onkologickych hlaseni a metodika prace onkologickeho oddenleni v okrese. Prakt. Lekar. 50, 3, 95-99 (1970).
12. LATOURETTE, H. B.: The use and value of tumor registry data. Amer. J. Roentgenol. 96, 1, 224-229 (1966).
13. NORA, P. F., VANECKO, R. M.: Method of peer review for cancer cure. Illinois Med. J. 140, 132-136 (1971).
14. OLSON, K. B., STONE, M., HARLAN, A.: The hospital tumor registry. Path. Ann. 5, 257-277 (1970).
15. PEDERSEN, E.: Some uses of the cancer registry in cancer control. Brit. J. Preventive & Social Medicine, April 1962, 16, 2.
16. SPRATT, J. S., JR.: The tumor registry - a definition. CA (N.Y.) 15, 3, 125-127 (1965).
17. VALK, Y.: The use of punchcards in cancer institutes. Vop.onkologii, 14, 1, 67-71 (1968).
18. WOLF-TERROINE, M.: Data processing in oncology. Methods of Information in Medicine. 5, 2, 60-67 (1966).
19. US Department of Health, Education and Welfare, Bethesda, Maryland Computers in design of hospital or medical facilities, Mid 1963-1966, 10 citations, L. S. No. 3-67.
20. UICC: Cancer Registries Symposium, 1970.
21. Seminar on Cancer Registries in Latin America, Cali, Colombia, 15-20 September 1969, Pan American Health Organization, Regional Office of the World Health Organization, 1970.

APPENDIX I

Justifications for and Aims of Hospital-Based Cancer Registries, as Collected from Different Literature Sources:

A) From the viewpoint of the cancer institute, or specialized departments of hospitals:

1. To furnish exact figures on the demand made on the facilities, personnel and resources of the institution by cancer patients, including changes in those demands with time, so as to establish a better basis for planning.
2. To give the total number of patients seen annually, categorized by site of cancer.
3. To show the trends in mortality in the area covered by the institute.
4. To show changes in the incidence and the age distribution in the area covered.
5. To show changes and trends in treatment modalities or policies with time
6. To show survival in general for different cancer sites.
7. To show survival in relation to the stage at admission.
8. To show survival in relation to treatment modalities and policies.
9. To provide in easily accessible form data that will facilitate a continuous search for problems that may require special research (e.g. in the form of clinical trials or epidemiological investigations).
10. To facilitate the follow-up of all patients for clinical purposes and for assessment of end results.
11. To show the number of primary lesions as compared with recurrent ones.
12. To facilitate identification and retrieval of particular data for research purposes.
13. To provide the physicians treating patients with a constantly up-to-date system of information on the current rate of accomplishment in their endeavor.
14. To allow crude evaluations: e.g.:
    a) are small tumors found?
    b) is in-situ cancer of the cervix searched for?
    c) has the prognosis (or survival) of malignant lymphoma been altered by supervoltage and more progressive therapy?
    d) has chemotherapy altered the survival time of patients with acute leukemia, or other malignancies etc.?
15. Hospital-based cancer registry is therefore to be considered as an organized attempt to offer an essential basis for the evaluation of current therapy with the effects of new treatment facilities, modalities, policies or management in the future.

B) From the aspect of the general cancer care situation and educational level in the area covered by the hospital cancer registry:

16. To record the number of cases diagnosed in this hospital compared with the number of cases first diagnosed elsewhere.
17. To allow calculation of the ratio between localized and advanced cases at the time of diagnosis and the change in this ratio year by year.
18. To record the lapse of time between the first symptoms and first therapy.

19. To record waiting time for admission to the hospital.
20. To record the duration of treatment or stay in hospital.
21. To provide information for population-based cancer registries.

C) For standardization or unification of hospital cancer registries:

22. To facilitate the exchange of information and of the organization of studies in collaboration with population-based cancer registries,where these exist, and with other hospital cancer registries at national or international level.
23. To furnish information for international cancer data banking system(s) if established in future.

Limitations:

1. The catchment area of an institution may overlap that of another.
2. The facilities existing in the institution may bias the "incidence".
3. The population at risk and morbidity data cannot be recorded adequately.
4. Only the ratio $\frac{\text{incidence}}{\text{mortality}}$ can give information on the effectiveness of cancer control measures.

APPENDIX II

Items of Information Coded in 26 Registries in Euro and Emro

A) Patient identification

Department of hospital		0/26
Record number		21/26
Personal identification number		5/26
Name of patient		
	Family name	25/26
	First name	23/26
Registration number		0/26
Address of patient		21/26
Sex		24/26
Date of birth		18/26
Civil status		10/26
	3 categories	9/26
	4 categories	10/26
	5 categories	3/26
Occupation		15/26
	6 categories	7/26
	5 categories	6/26
Nationality		6/26
Religion		3/26
Race		0/26
Place of birth		8/26
Hospital registry number		0/26
Income level	3 categories	4/26
Age group		17/26

B) Patient history

Item		Count
Date of first diagnosis of present cancer		
	Diagnosis at admission (ICD)	21/26
	Clinical diagnosis & data (ICD)	20/26
	Cytological diagnosis and date	10/26
	Histopathologic diagnosis and date	23/26
Previous treatment		12/26
Date of first symptoms (year, month)		12/26
Age at first diagnosis		0/26
Delay between first symptoms and first specific treatment		0/26
	a) delay between first symptom and check-up	12/26
	b) delay between check-up and admission to hospital	9/26
Number of children		6/26
Number of miscarriages		5/26
Stillbirths		3/26
Number of pregnancies		2/26
Menstrual history		6/26
Age at menarche		5/26
Age at menopause		3/26
Cancer in descendants		5/26
Cancer in ascendants		4/26
Cancer in blood relatives		5/26
Exposure to potential carcinogens		5/26
3 categories of pollution of workingenvironment		1/26
Abuse of alcohol and nicotine		3/26
Eating habits and food composition		1/26
Accidents		2/26
Other simultaneous (chronic) disease		2/26
Height		2/26
Weight		3/26
Precanceroses		4/26
Coded descriptions of environment		1/26
Previous important or chronic disease		7/26

C) Present disease

Item		Count
Date of first admission to hospital		16/26
Primary site		17/26
Mode of diagnosis		0/26
Histological type		23/26
Tumor stage at first admission		14/26
Tumor stage at first admission if TNM is not applicable		14/26
Simultaneous primary tumors		6/26
Treatment in hospital		
Surgery		19/26
X-ray		20/26
Drug therapy		19/26
Other forms of therapy		19/26
Duration of hospitalization		3/26
Status at discharge		8/26
Age at first admission to hospital		17/26
Disease status		8/26
Sites of metastases		14/26
Notification of population-based registry		12/26
Further details of treatment		
	1. Surgery	5/26

2. Radiotherapy	13/26
3. Chemotherapy	6/26
4. Hormone therapy	0/26
5. Other	0/26
No treatment	8/26
Curative treatment	14/26
Palliative treatment	14/26
Metastases (not giving the site)	16/26
Secondary nodes	14/26
Intercurrent complications	1/26
Combined therapies	7/26
Duration of treatment	3/26
Complications of treatment	2/26
Sequence and numbers of therapies and dates	12/26

D) Follow-up

Date of next follow-up	8/26
Status at follow-up	8/26

E) Death

Date of death	16/26
Cause of death	8/26
Performance of autopsy	16/26
Incidental cancer found at autopsy	0/26
Survival	11/26

F) Other

Discrepancy between clinical and pathologic or postmortem diagnosis	2/26
Place of death	4/26
Death unrelated to cancer	6/26
Name of hospital	20/26
Anniversary dates	6/26
Name of accepting physician	12/26
Name of therapist	5/26
Name of registrar	5/26
Blood group	2/26
Invalidization, incapacitation	2/26

The Collection of Available Information: Possibilities and Limitations of International Standardization

A. J. Tuyns

1. Introduction: Definition of the Subject

For the epidemiologist, one of the main objectives of cancer registries is to establish accurate incidence data for the various types of cancer and thus to allow comparison from region to region. When differences become apparent these can then be used as bases for hypotheses and for etiological studies.

However, such comparisons are only possible if the data are comparable and thus if sufficient care to ensure comparability has been taken during the successive stages of the work.

These various stages are listed in Table 1, together with methods used to improve comparability for each stage. Great progress has been made towards the standardization of coding methods, data processing, and presentation of results. Epidemiological methods allowing better comparability are available for analysis of the results.

Table 1. Cancer Registration. Standardization

0.	Medical identification of cancer cases Generation of information	
1.	Collection and verification of information	
2.	Data processing	
	-coding	Codes WHO, MOTNAC ... Standardization of coding procedures
	-transcription onto cards, tapes, etc.	Standardization of techniques
	-tabulation	Standardization of tables (cf. CI5C)
3.	Analysis of results	Epidemiological methods of analysis

The first steps of the work, i.e. the actual collection and verification of information, have not received the same amount of attention. The purpose of this paper is to describe and discuss the disparity of methods used at this level and to suggest either standardization, whenever this is possible, or alternative measures.

2. Collection of Information

The medical route followed by a cancer patient during the course of his illness may vary considerably from one region to another, because of the different medical structures and habits. Even within the same region the pathways may vary depending on the type of cancer or the personal behavior of the patient. The information relevant to the patient is scattered in many different places, all of which must be considered as potential sources of information by the cancer registry.

Sources of Information

In a given region, all hospitals or clinics and all doctors are likely to see patients with cancer, and should theoretically be used as sources of information. In practice this is never done and only selected sources are systematically explored.

Among the registries which provided data for the book on Cancer Incidence in Five Continents, there was a considerable amount of variation in the respective contributions from major types of sources of information. The percentage of cases discovered from death certificates only varied from 0 to 20% while the contribution of pathology laboratories varied from 0 to 60%. There were extreme situations where the registry only recorded cases from cancer centers or even only some of them (e.g. those confirmed by pathology). It is usually stated that "all" cancer patients in the area pass through these centers, which is probably wishful thinking. A few examples of contribution patterns are shown in Fig. 1.

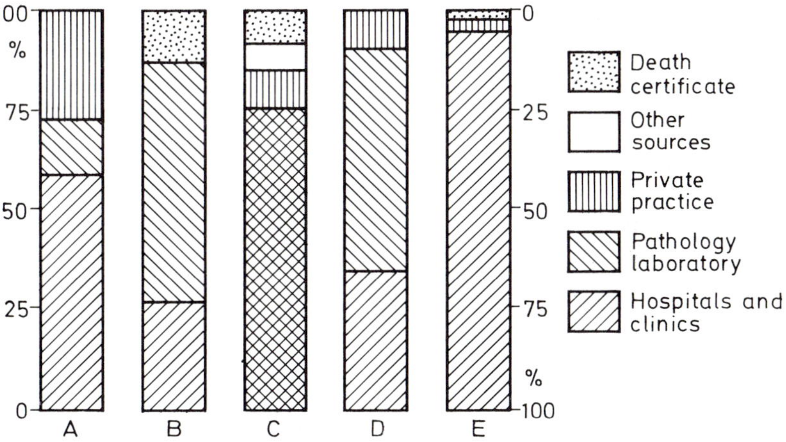

Fig. 1. Sources of information in five cancer registries

There is, of course, room for subjective interpretation of such data. A contribution "nil" by death certificates might indicate that all reported deaths were for patients already notified and thus known to the registry. Often, it means that mortality data have not been used or that there is no death registration at all in the area.

In spite of its relative imprecision, such information seems nevertheless to indicate a great diversity in the use of sources of information in the existing registries, raising serious doubts as to the complete recording of certain categories of cancer patients and the comparability of data recorded.

Every registry, of course, operates in a given medical framework which is a de-facto situation which cannot be altered. In this respect, standardization is out of the question. What a registry can and should do, however, is to keep a complete list of the potential sources of information and a listing of their informants; any exclusion of a source should be justified. This may imply ad hoc sampling surveys.

Type of Information Requested

In the various kinds of questionnaires used in cancer registries, there is a great diversity in the type of information sought; nevertheless, there is a common background of basic items in most of them. These are used in the basic tabulations needed for comparisons.

This apparent resemblance may in fact hide differences of significant importance. The method of ascertaining the religious or ethnic group may not be equally reliable everywhere. A given "residence" or even a given "age" is likely to have a different meaning in London and Ibadan. For items such as "occupation" or belonging to an "urban" or "rural" zone, there is an even greater risk to deal with, interpretation of these concepts being sometimes radically different.

The registries which contributed to Cancer Incidence in Five Continents used substantially different definitions of the starting point of the cancer, which was used as an index date for the classification of patients by year of incidence (Table 2).

Table 2. Dates used as "Date of Onset" of Cancer for Records of Cancer Incidence

Date of first symptom.
Date of suspicion of cancer.
Date of first medical examination.
Date of admission to the hospital for the illness subsequently diagnosed as cancer; failing this, date of biopsy, failing this, date of death.
Date of diagnosis.
Date of first definitive diagnosis.
Date of histological diagnosis; for those not confirmed by histology, date of admission to hospital.
Date of first treatment, or date of admission to hospital if not treated.
Date of discharge from hospital, or date of death.
Date of recording.
Case history.

A minimum list of items to be recorded could easily be drawn up and agreed upon by all registries. For more detailed specific points each registry should be free to incorporate those they feel they can use.

It is more important to obtain from each registry the definitions of the terms and the classifications used, even for simple things like age, residence and profession, than to standardize questionnaires.

International agreement can probably be reached on the definition and use of certain items such as "index date," for which proposals have already been formulated. Similar arrangements could perhaps be made for "residence," which could, for example, be the place where the patient had actually lived during at least six months before his illness; the "occupation" recorded could be the last one before the onset of the disease.

3. Checking of the Information Received

The information is checked partly at the registry itself and partly at the place of collection. The methods used in the verification of completeness, consistency, etc. are discussed elsewhere. Only some facts which might influence comparability are mentioned here.

The most obvious seems to be the tracing of duplicates, which is based essentially on the similarity of certain identification elements appearing in the notifications registered at different times and derived from different sources. Usually the name, sex, date of birth, and place of residence are used. These items are extremely precious when they are both accurate and stable. When, for example, such essential items as name and age are unusable, tracing duplicates becomes a more difficult job; additional items have to be taken into account and even then decisions are difficult.

Depending upon the severity of the reviser, elimination of duplicates may or may not be drastic, leading to deflation of inflation of the number of cases.

Checking procedures cannot be fully standardized but the problem should be looked into; minimum requirements for checking should be recommended, bearing in mind that computerization can help but only to a certain extent.

4. The Medical and Clinical Structure - the Information Actually Available

The task of a cancer registry is to seek all the available information on cancer cases, to register them and to analyze them. This ideal mass of information - the maximum available - is closely linked to both the number and the quality of the medical and clinical facilities available in the area.

Quality of medicine cannot be easily compared from one area to another. Incompetence leading to erroneous diagnosis is probably neither more frequent nor more confusing than the over-refinement which leads to the over-recording of certain cases (e.g. cancer *in situ*, "borderline" cases).

The quantitative aspect, in contrast, is simple to evaluate. Amongst the registries whose data were published in Cancer Incidence in Five Continents, the number of doctors per 1,000 inhabitants varied from 0.2 to 2.6, and the number of hospital beds per 1,000 inhabitants from 1.2 to 13.0. Cases are more likely to be missed in some situation than others. Such omissions are often selective.

Under-registration connected with lack of medical personnel is particularly noticeable in Africa, where the arrival or the departure of one doctor can completely upset the reported picture of cancer in a given area.

In one country of 900 000 inhabitants, only one case of cancer of the ovary was found in 1965; in 1966, there were 11, due to the arrival of a competent gynecologist.
In another country, amongst the four major ethnic groups, only one showed a high frequency of bronchial carcinoma (5.9% of cancers), contrasting with 0.9 to 2.6% in the other ethnic groups; it turned out to be the group attended by the only chest surgeon in the country.

These rather caricatural examples are given to illustrate the kind of distortions that probably occur elsewhere in a less spectacular way. Even under the most favorable conditions, the lack of a sufficient number of neurosurgeons, of urologists or other specialists, or their reluctance to collaborate with the cancer registry can produce selective under-reporting for certain tumors.

There is no real remedy for such situations, but as has been said above, a registry must at least be able to give the number of available specialists in the area covered and report how many of them collaborate efficiently by notification of cancer cases they see.

Discussion

Epidemiologists require comparable data that is clear of undesirable biases. They are right in proposing as great a degree of standardization as is possible in order to obtain this end. There is, however, a certain limit to be worked towards, which must not be passed beyond. As long as standardization entails imposing rules which would affect only comfort, ease, or liberty of the registrars, it is permissible. When facts and situations have to be distorted to fit uniform definitions, standardization is no longer legitimate.

In the first stages of cancer registration, there are methods that lend themselves to uniformity and they must be standardized. There are also differences in concepts which cannot be standardized but can and must be carefully defined in each registry. There are, finally, facts and situations over which we have no control and which also need to be defined.

Only some of these differences have been mentioned in this brief outline, and a more detailed and thorough analysis is obviously needed. It is the responsibility of the registries themselves to start this introspective and autocritical work. Assistance from outside is desirable and even indispensable. Particulars that vary from region to region are only visible from the outside; to the inside observer they look simply "normal" and "obvious". This delicate evaluation must be performed by independent international organizations with due respect for individual and national susceptibilities. The International Association of Cancer Registries and the International Agency for Research on Cancer are prepared to assist in this work.

Production of data for the use of the epidemiologists is not the sole objective of a cancer registry. It is also a tool for national or regional public health purposes, regardless of any international uses, and this must not be underestimated.

The danger of international perfectionism must not be overlooked. It is tempting to take as examples registries which are working well in certain areas and try to promote their methods in other regions where medical structures may be radically different and hence chances of success remote. This might lead to the development of overstandardized registries only in areas that are similar in their medicosocial patterns (e.g. in a few so-called developed countries) where true environmental differences are unlikely to vary to any considerable extent. From the epidemiological viewpoint it is far more important to have more new registries in other parts of the world.

Most cancer registries had to start with a limited scheme, and the progressive inclusion of more new sources, more information, and improvements came later, leading eventually to a full-scale population-based cancer registration scheme - a stage which few registries can yet claim to have reached.

Standardization must be increased and improved within reasonable limits but care must be taken not to discourage new attempts in countries with widely differing medical facilities and patterns which require understanding and imagination.

The ideal complete cancer registry cannot be achieved at once; limited but realistic schemes are admissible and desirable. Excessive standardization might inhibit such initiatives, and epidemiology would be the loser.

References

TUYNS, A.: Techniques of Registration. In: Cancer Incidence in Five Continents, Vol. 2. UICC 1970.

WHO: Expert Committee on Health Statistics. Third Report, including Second Report of the Sub-Committee on Cancer Statistics. WHO Tech. Report Ser. 53, 1952.

WHO: Expert Committee on Health Statistics. Sixth Report, including Third Report of the Sub-Committee on Cancer Statistics. WHO Tech. Report Ser. 164, 1959.

Problems in the Initiation of a Cancer Registry

E. Anglesio*

Introduction

The aim of creating tumor registries was the improvement of the approach to problems relevant to cancer. Increased knowledge of the frequency of malignant diseases, their distribution, incidence, and mortality is of primary importance for cancer control, and the relevant figures can only be obtained through registries. Good registration demands adequate organization in many spheres, as suggested by our own experience.

Liaison with outside Organizations

Good contacts must be developed, primarily with governmental health departments, to obtain authorization to collect data within the framework of a regional or national cancer program. These departments must inform the hospitals in the area of this program and of the need for registration of new tumor cases (Fig. 1).

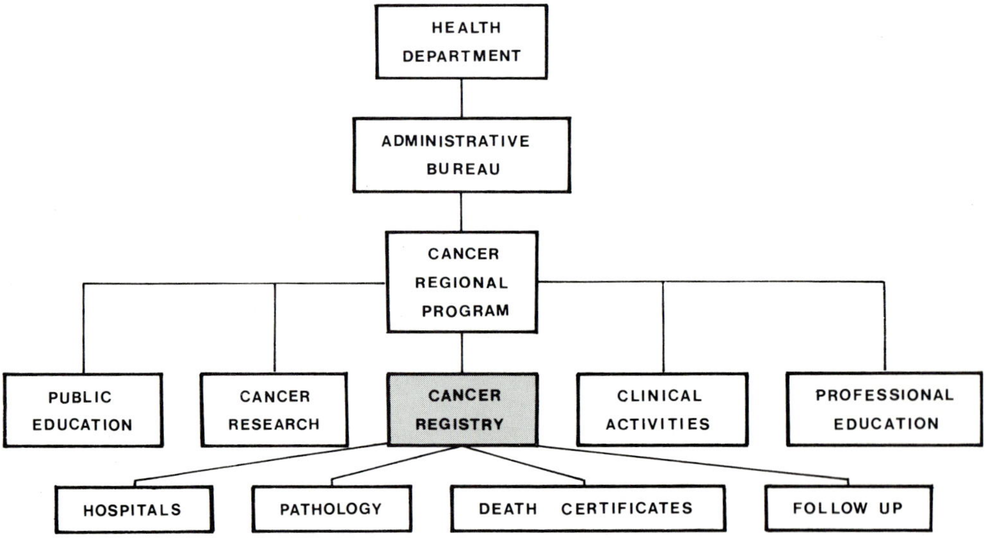

Fig. 1

*Registro dei Tumori per il Piemonte e la valle d'Aosta-Torino

It is not always easy to persuade health officers that the patterns of malignant diseases vary according to multiple factors such as geographical position, occupation, life-style, food, and ages of various populations (as emphasized by epidemiological observations over the last 30 years). Administrative and health officers should be aware that the initiative of starting a registry may actively contribute to professional and public education.
The health department must inform the administrative bureau about the program because of the financial planning. Allocation of a budget is an extremely confusing task in view of the current fall in the value of money and the increasing cost of personnel. Both present and future needs must be considered and costs must be estimated for a period of five years at least.

Financial resources must be related to the size of the registry, and this depends on the cancer caseload.
The cost of a registry includes the following items (Table 1):

Table 1. Financing

Financing
1 - Advisory board time
2 - Salary of personnel for routine operations
3 - Office space and furniture
4 - General routine fees (mail, telephone, etc.)
5 - Special stationery (forms, sheets, etc.)
6 - Books, codes, manuals
7 - Cost of abstracts, whether obtained from hospitals or prepared by own abstractors
8 - Computerizing and data processing
9 - Travel to visits and meetings

The current cost calculated by the California tumor registry is about $ 10.00 per new case, but may be more.

According to the experience of the Connecticut and California tumor registries, the cancer caseload is about 3.2 to 3.0 percent of admissions to hospitals (Ringel). Immich, in Heidelberg, calculated 3.56%.

Special agreements have to be reached with hospitals so that the abstractors can have access to patient charts and records or consignments of abstracts of patient records be sent periodically.

Arrangements should be made with pathology institutions so that reports of all tumors submitted for histological and cytological examinations can be obtained even if they are not included in hospital abstracts. An agreement must also be maintained with the Registrar of births and deaths so that a list of deaths with the causes of death be sent periodically.

The professional Council should be contacted so that all physicians can be acquainted with the objectives and purposes of registration and collaborate more carefully in following cancer patients and filling in the questionnaires with due care.

For these liaisons to be successfull an Advisory Board or Committee must be created, comprising (Table 2):

Table 2. Advisory Board

Advisory Board
1 - Representative of the governmental health department
2 - Director of the Regional Cancer Program
3 - Representative of the administrative bureau
4 - Hospital representative
5 - Representative of the professional Council
6 - Director of the Registry

The task of the Advisory Board is the periodic appraisal of the policy and practical matters related to registration.

Internal Organization

Staff. The staff should include (Table 3) a director (an oncologist), a pathologist, a statistician, an epidemiologist, and an administrator. The staff should meet regularly to discuss various problems and to establish the philosophy of registration (e.g. what cases are to be registered).

Table 3. Staff

Staff
1 - Executive officer (Director)
2 - Epidemiologist
3 - Pathologist
4 - Statistician
5 - Administrator

Personnel (Table 4). The scarcity of people trained in statistics and epidemiology makes the choice of good personnel rather difficult. It is probably best to employ people already engaged in hospital work. New personnel must be trained in statistical methodology, medical terminology, coding facilities, and preparation of reports.

Table 4. Personnel

Personnel
1 - Staff members
2 - Secretary
3 - Coders
4 - Abstractor clerks
5 - Archivist
6 - Ancillary personnel

Special short-term courses should be established for abstractors or hospital clerks to train them in the techniques of accurate abstracting and coding (often from inadequate medical charts or incomplete records). These people must receive continuous guidance and assistance in order to ensure high standards and uniformity in completion of the registration sheets.

Documents (Table 5). There are many kinds of questionnaires in use and this makes the choice difficult. Registration sheets must be simple, clear, and complete. A bulk of unnecessary data is disturbing. Most sheets contain core data and optional data.

Table 5. Documents

Documents
1 - Registration forms
2 - Pathology reports
3 - Death certificates
4 - Follow-up sheets
5 - Master file cards
6 - Envelope or binding for archives

The information most frequently requested falls into three categories:

1) identification and personal data,
2) pathological data, and
3) treatment and follow-up.

These are core data; optional data can be added in forms.

Pathology reports can be obtained directly from pathology institutions.

Death certificates are supplied at monthly intervals by the Registrar of births and deaths.

Follow-up sheets include a questionnaire to be sent to the treating hospitals or physicians. The questions must be limited to very brief data concerning the status of patients.

Master file. An alphabetic master file must be prepared. The charts in this file must contain a minimum of data for the identification of patients.

When the charts arrive at the registry, each document must be checked by the personnel and questionnaires and sheets must be matched with pathology reports, lists of deaths, and follow-up sheets and matched with the master file. For new cases the data must be completed and numbers allocated, and for known ones the documents are retrieved for the addition of new information; all the information is then coded.

Processing (Fig. 2). When the coded sheets have been completed in every section they are ready for processing and are sent for punching. The data recorded on the punched cards must be stored on magnetic tape or in some other way suitable for processing. At this stage the registry has achieved the first of its objectives.

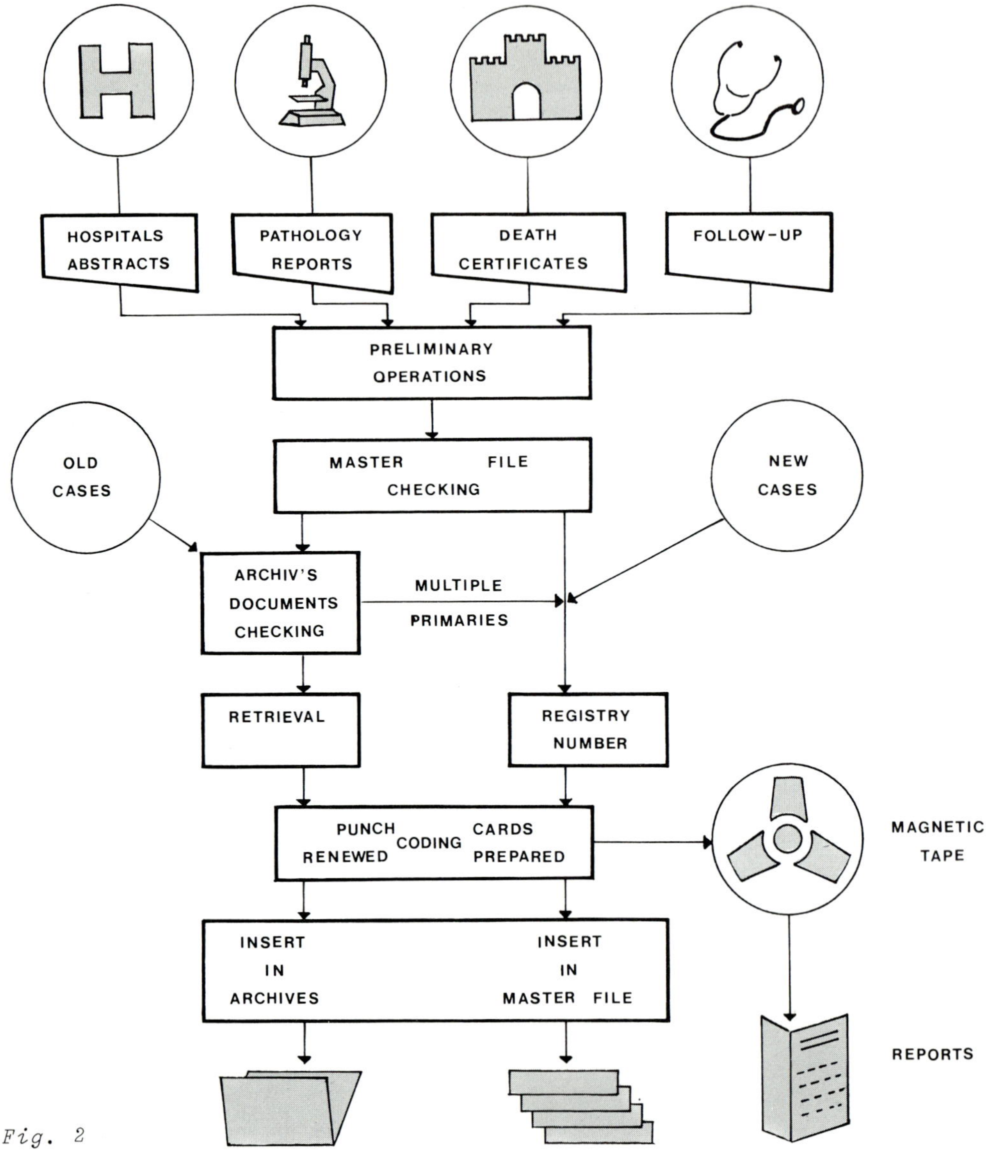

Fig. 2

Utilization. The computer system is periodically requested to print out the data in tabulated form to allow the preparation of annual reports on numbers of cases, percentages, incidence and distribution by sex and age. These reports must be sent to health departments, hospitals, registries, and physicians; they document the activity and full potential of the registry.

Archives. All the documents mentioned must be kept in special boxes or archives sorted both alphabetically and by anatomical site. Since all information cannot be coded simultaneously, in the case of special requests for individual studies the charts must be at hand for further use. In the case of retrieval, new data can be introduced or modified, e.g. for long survival.

Special Problems

Adequate quality control of the data must be checked routinely at regular intervals. Accuracy in abstracting and coding is the only criterion for the availability of the registry data. These must be completed by histological and cytological results, follow-up data and/or death certificates.

Experience thus far has established that ratios of new cases to cases lost to death are estimated at 1.6 to 1.

Good registration will be impossible if, the apathy of administrators, hospitals, and physicians is not overcome. They should be persuaded that knowledge of the epidemiological patterns of tumors is a good way to improve both diagnosis and treatment of tumors.

The Computerized Registry

A. Barnes, P.M. Payne and R.G. Skeet

1. The South Metropolitan Cancer Registry

It would be impossible to give a full account of the different ways in which a computer can be used to advantage in a cancer registry. This paper is therefore restricted to the computer system used at the South Metropolitan Cancer Registry.

Understanding of this computer system requires some knowledge of the structure of the Registry and the way in which it functions. Fig. 1 is a simplified representation of the cancer registry and its main lines of communication. On the left are the Registry's three main sources of data, the hospitals, the patients' general practitioners and the Office of Population Censuses and Surveys, which provides copies of death certificates. In the center are the four internal departments of the Registry; the registration department, the coding department, the data preparation and handling department and the follow-up department; and on the right is the computer bureau.

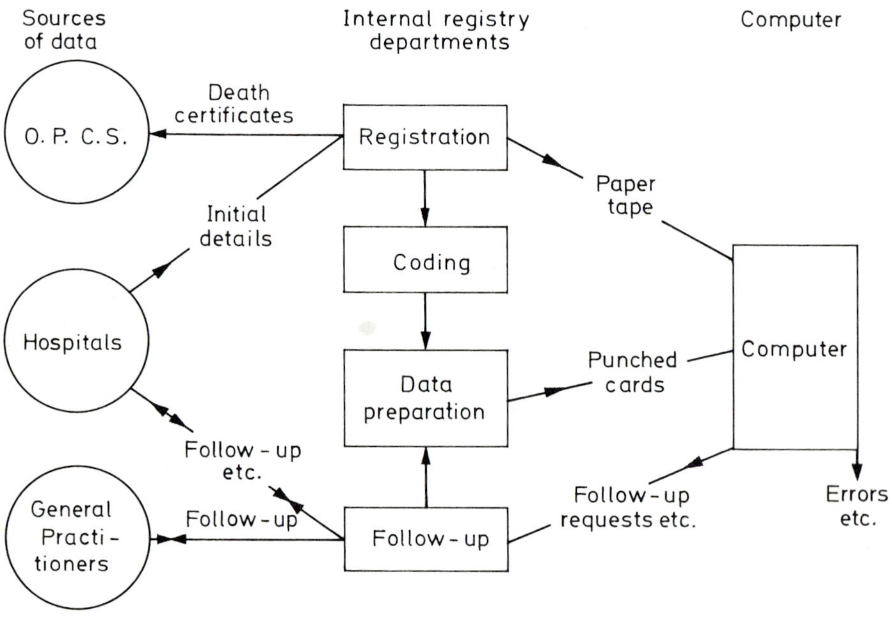

Fig. 1. Diagram of the S. M. C. R. & main lines of communication

The Registry is initially notified of a case of cancer in one of two ways. In approximatley 90% of cases a completed registration form is received from one of a number of clerks employed by the Registry to abstract data from hospital case notes. A second method of notification is the receipt of a death certificate followed by enquiries either to a hospital or to the patient's general practitioner if the patient did not die in hospital.

On receipt at the cancer registry,all the completed registration forms are initially dealt with by the registration department. The patient's details are checked against a phonetic index of all registered cases to ensure that the tumor is not already registered and to increase the probability of finding patients with more than one primary cancer. If the tumor is not yet registered a registration number is allocated and the patient's name, address and diagnosis are punched into paper tape. It will be seen later that this paper tape is an important part of the computer system. A small card, also containing the patient's name, address and diagnosis, is typed as a by-product of the paper tape and is immediately filed into the phonetic index, thus keeping the index up to date at all times.

Following the production of the paper tape the registration form is passed on to the coding department. This department is concerned mainly with the translation of information on the registration form into codes so that it can be readily punched into cards for subsequent computer input. The actual coding process is probably very similar to that used by any other cancer registry. When the coding is completed, the registration form is filed away and the completed coding forms passed on to the data preparation department, where the coded information is punched into 80-column computer cards. When punched, the cards are grouped into batches of between 1000 and 2000 cards for handling and identification purposes and are then ready for input to the computer.

It is in the follow-up department that the system has been found to be most helpful. This department deals with all requests for further information about registered cancer cases. It also deals with requests for details of postmortem examinations carried out on registered patients. A further function of the department is to notify hospitals of the deaths of its cancer patients.

2. The Computer Record

The Registry's computer system uses magnetic tape as its storage medium. The reasons for this are partly historical and partly due to the amount of data to be stored, which is large even by computer standards. The cancer patient records are held in registration number order on one of two magnetic tape files, the "live master file" and the "dead master file." The "live master file" contains all the records of patients who are still alive and also contains a proportion of records relating to patients who have died recently. The "dead master file" holds the remaining records of dead cases. The reason for this division will become apparent later.

Fig. 2 illustrates a record as it is held on the magnetic tape. The record is divided into a number of sections, each of which corresponds to one type of information about the tumor. The three sections of the record following the registration number, dealing with clinical history, treatment, and hospitals attended, hold information that is usually coded by the coding department from the initial registration form.

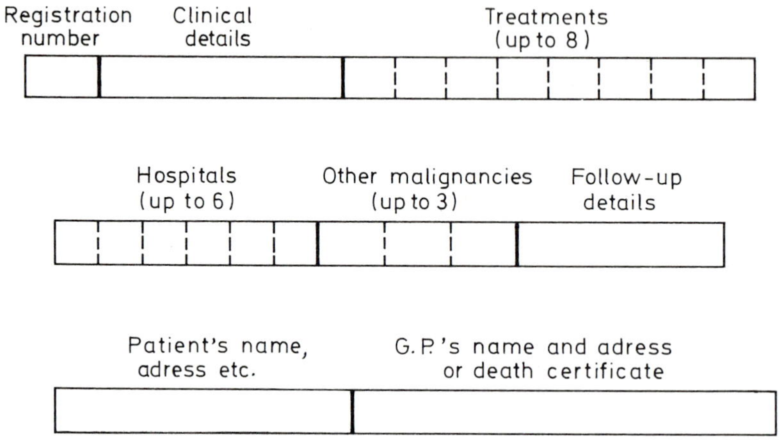

Fig. 2. The record as held on magnetic tape

The other malignancies section will contain information only when the patient is known to have one or more additional primary cancers. The section relating to follow-up is empty until either result of the first year follow-up or notification of death is received. The final section of the record contains either the general practitioner's name and address or the details on the death certificate, depending on whether the patient is alive or dead. Within a few months of being notified of the patient's death this section of the record is removed, resulting in a significant reduction in the length of the computer record.

The paper tape produced in the registration department is the initial input for the computer for each case. When it is read, a full-length record is set on the magnetic tape but at this point, other parts of the record are almost completely empty. Data relating to all the other sections are fed into the computer on punched cards. These punched cards are distinguished by the "input-type" number which appears at the beginning of each card and which identifies one particular section of the record. The registration number which identifies the record itself is always the next piece of information on the card and this is followed by the first three letters of the patient's surname. (These letters serve as a precaution against incorrect transcription of the registration number and this or a similar check has been found to be very important). The information to be input to the record follows after this part of the card.

A very important part of this system is the procedure used to amend or add information to a section of a record that already contains information. Corresponding to each section of the computer record, in addition to the initial "input-type," there is an amendment form with which it is possible to change or add any piece of information in that section

3. Updating the Files

Every month all paper tape and punched cards produced over the previous thirty days are collected together and fed into the computer to up-date the live master file (Fig. 3).

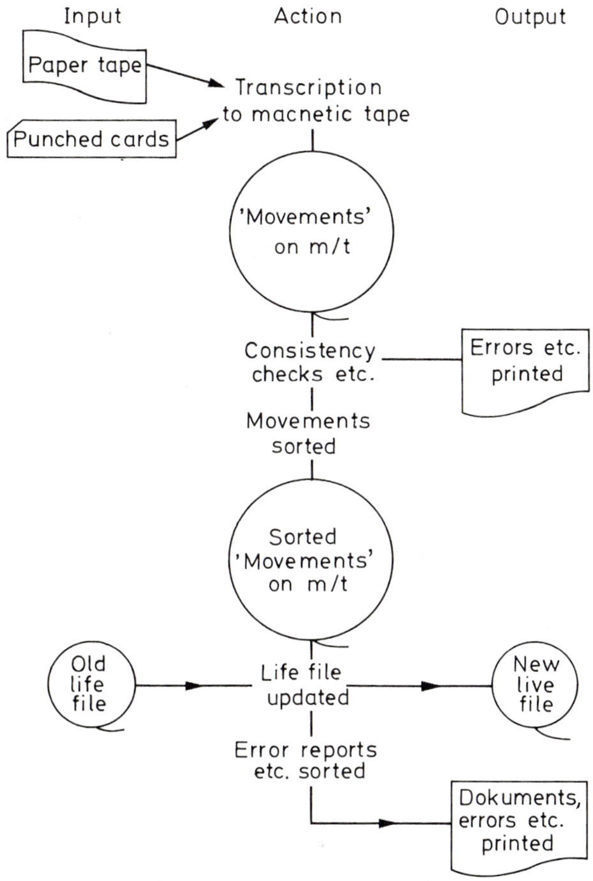

Fig. 3. Updating the live master file

The first part of the process consists in the transfer of all the data on all the paper tape and punched cards onto magnetic tape. The image of a paper tape record or a punched card as it is held on the magnetic tape is referred to as a "movement." At this point, the ordering of the movements is entirely immaterial.Following their transcription to magnetic tape a number of checks are applied to the information contained in the movements. These checks are concerned mainly with the consistency of the information and with ensuring that the codes fall within admissible ranges of values. Movements which fail one or more of these checks are listed with details of the error. The accepted movements are then sorted into registration number order and are read in parallel with the old version of the live master file.

Where a movement registration number matches a record on the master file, the movement is used to update or amend that record, but before this is done further consistency checks are carried out on the information which would result from updating the record. Movements which pass these further checks are incorporated into the record in a way that is dependent on the movement type and those that fail are listed as before.

When all movements have been dealt with for a particular record an examination is carried out to see whether any documents or messages are to be produced for the record. Four different types of documents can be produced, viz.:

1) a request for follow-up information from a hospital,
2) a request for follow-up information from a general practitioner,
3) a request for details of any postmortem findings, and
4) a document giving details from the death certificate.

A follow-up request is produced for each live patient on every anniversary of his first treatment, and a 'Flag' in the record determines where the request for information should be sent. A request for postmortem information is produced whenever a patient is known to have died in a hospital. The document giving details of the death certificate is produced as soon as the record receives this information. One of these documents is printed and sent to each hospital attended by the patient other than the hospital in which he died.

These documents are preprinted forms to which the computer adds certain details such as the name and address of the patient, hospital case number, etc. An example of one of these forms, the death notification form, is given in Figs.4, 5.

Notification of Death
S. M. C. R., Clifton Avenue, Belmont, Sutton, Surrey

Date

Case No. Hospital Consultants

We have recently been informed that on
the death of the undermentioned patient occurred:

Surname Forenames	Address

Cause of Death:

Ia
b
c
II

Place of Death

P. M. Done
P. M. Payne
Director

Fig. 4. Example of preprinted form

In addition to these preprinted documents, a number of administrative lists and messages can be printed by the computer. One of these gives a complete listing of the contents of a record and can be requested when the contents of the computer record are in doubt. When all the messages, documents, etc. have been printed, the updated record is added to the new live master file and the next record is considered. This process is continued until all the records have been transferred to the new master file. When the updating is completed the documents printed by the computer are sent out by the follow-up department. The lists and messages are dealt with by the data handling department where the errors are investigated and corrected.Corrections are added to the next live master file up-date.

Notification of Death
S. M. C. R., Clifton Avenue, Belmont, Sutton, Surrey
Date 25/02/73

Case No.	Hospital	Consultants
69/46541	St. Ruth's	M179 M 106

We have recently been informed that on 19 Dec. 1972
the death of the undermentioned patient occurred:

Surname	Williams	Address	4 Bunkers Hill,
Forenames	Thomas Stanley		Denmead,
			Surrey

Cause of Death:

Ia congestive cardiac failure
b mitral stenosis
c Oat cell carcinoma lung
II

Place of Death Home P. M. Done Yes

P. M. Payne
Director

Fig. 5. Example of preprinted form with computer additions

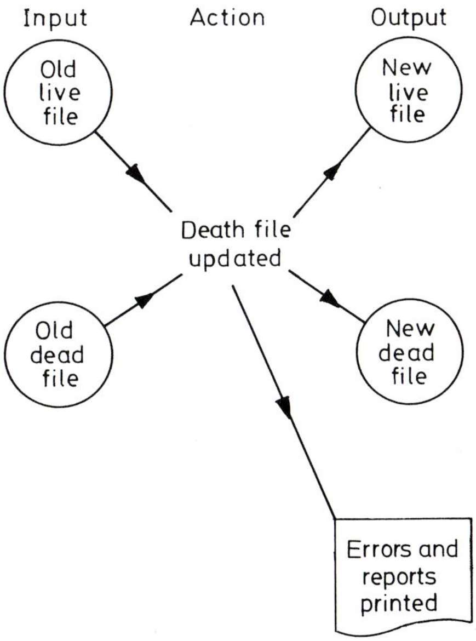

Fig. 6. Updating the dead master file

The dead master file is updated once every four months (Fig. 6) and this process is somewhat simpler. The number of dead cancer cases soon becomes larger than the number of live cases and this is why it is considered essential to have separate live and dead master files. If this were not done, updating of the live master file would be a very much slower process because of the very large number of records (relating to dead patients) for which few changes or additions are likely. In fact, the main purpose of updating the dead master file is to transfer from the live file all those records which have been closed due to notification of death in the previous four months. It is also during this transfer that the length of the record is reduced by removal of the final section of the record. It is still possible to add or change information contained in a record relating to a dead patient. This is done by feeding in information to the live master file up-date on the appropriate punched card. The information on the card is then held on the live file to await the next dead up-date when the amendment takes place.

This computer system has now been in use for slightly more than three years and has been found to be quite successful. Most of the problems there have been have resulted from technical trouble with the computer itself and most of them occurred soon after the system was introduced. Finally, this system was specifically designed to meet the requirements and circumstances of the South Metropolitan Cancer Registry. Other cancer registries have their own requirements and circumstances and would probably find parts of this system impractical or unnecessary.

The Ninth Revision of ICD Chapter on Neoplasms and its Application in Oncology

H. Tulinius

This paper deals with ICD(9) and ICD(O), the second chapter of the ninth revision of the International Classification of Diseases, which deals with neoplasms and its application in oncology. The proposals for the 9th revision are still in the preparatory stages, and will be subjected to further review. Whether there will be changes between now and adoption of the revision by the General Assembly of the World Health Organization (WHO) is not certain. The information in this paper is based on the proposals and on the assumption that they will be accepted.

The International Classification of Diseases, Injuries and Causes of Death, to give its full name, has of late been revised approximately every 10 years, and since the WHO came into being it has been responsible for its preparation, revision, and publication. The revision in effect today is the 8th revision; this came into effect on 1 January 1968 (1). It is proposed that the 9th revision will be effective from 1 January 1978. WHO plans to have the printed tabular lists, indexes, etc., produced in 1976, and 1977 can then be used by Statistical Offices and other users of the ICD to prepare for its use from 1 January 1978 onward.

There has been a substantial amount of criticism of the changes introduced with the 8th revision, or more particularly of the chapter on cancer.

Any change in ICD is a very serious matter. This is partly because people who use it memorize the rubric numbers so that any change in these numbers is a source of error, but probably a more serious reason is that when changes are made, not only the numbers but also the contents of rubrics may change, and also their coding rules and definitions. For this reason, material coded under one ICD revision may not be comparable with the material coded according to the next revision. This leads to loss of continuity in health statistics and irreparable damage may be done.

Another area of criticism, which may be more important, is that the 8th revision did not promote much progress in the handling of data concerning the biological behavior of tumors.

One often hears of "the cancer problem" in the singular. This is very misleading because the neoplastic diseases are many. Traditional cancer epidemiology, which to some extent has been governed by the structure of ICD, has separated the malignant diseases into cancers arising in different organs. It is a step forward not to think of "the cancer problem" and to start thinking of the problem of neoplasms of individual organs, but only a step, since among the cancers arising in a single organ there may be many diseases. The next step seems to be the separation of the cancers into their morphological types. A fuller discussion of this is given in Dr. SAXÉN'S article in this volume.

This kind of criticism had reached the ears of the members of the Study Group for the 9th revision of the ICD, the WHO Group which determines policy for the revision as a whole. At their meeting in 1970 they decided that the 9th revision should be a conservative one, as while they felt a radical revision was called for, they considered that the time was not yet ripe for adequate preparation of such a radical revision; hence they decided to have the world wait for a radical 10th revision.

The International Agency for Research on Cancer had solicited the opinions of many workers in the field of cancer epidemiology and submitted some ideas to this Study Group meeting. As a result, the Study Group asked IARC to prepare a proposal for the neoplasms chapter of the 9th revision. This mandate included revision of rubric contents and the introduction of more 4th digits, and also the addition of a method for the coding of morphological type.

IARC decided to attack this problem from two angles. The correspondence with people interested in cancer epidemiology was continued and increased, which included soliciting the opinions of cancer registry workers, people in the health statistics offices of various countries, oncologically minded clinicians, cancer hospitals, etc. IARC then appointed two working parties,[1] one to handle the revision of rubric numbers, rubric contents, and the introduction of 4th digits, and the second to introduce a coding method for morphological type.

These two working parties made a joint proposal, which was put forward to the WHO Study Group that met in 1971. This proposal introduced a few changes in the handling of rubrics 140-199 and a number of new 4th digits, and it suggested the abolition of rubrics 200-239.

The neoplasms chapter (Chap. 2) of ICD(8) is divided into several fields. The biggest field, 140-199, handles the malignant neoplasms of organs other than the reticuloendothelial organs, and 200-209 embraces neoplasms of the reticuloendothelial organs. Rubrics 210-229 deal with benign tumors, and 230-239 other variously defined tumors including carcinoma in situ. Each of these fields is defined roughly on an anatomical basis, this principle being best developed in the largest field, i.e. that of malignant tumors of organs other than the reticuloendothelial organs.

The IARC working parties came to the conclusion that it was wasteful to separate a chapter into several fields with anatomical axes of varying degrees of precision, and that it would be better to use one fairly elaborate anatomical axis. It was therefore proposed that, instead of this separation of the chapter on cancer into fields, one digit be used to indicate the behavior of neoplastic disease. This was not an original idea, but was taken over from SNOP (Systematized Nomenclature of Pathology), which was introduced by the American College of Pathologists in 1965. The SNOP idea had then been taken and carried forward by the American Cancer Society when they produced MOTNAC (Manual of Tumor Nomenclature and Coding) in 1968. The argument in favor of this step is that if anatomical precision is needed for malignant neoplasms there is no reason why the same anatomical precision is not needed for benign neoplasms or for carcinomas in situ, etc. In addition, coding of morphological type involves some problems in selection of the exact "field." In some tumors the morphology is not

[1] C. S. MUIR, H. PAGE, E. PEDERSEN, E. SAXEN, L. SOBIN, H. TULINIUS, G. WAGNER, A. WINKLER.

decisive in the decision as to whether they are malignant or benign. There are also clinical conditions where it is not known whether the biopsy specimen is from a primary or a metastatic tumor. Problem cases of this kind would need to be relegated to single rubrics if the field approach were maintained, and hence all the information on anatomy and morphology would be lost.

In its deliberations on morphological type coding, the Working Party considered approximately 10 codes currently in use in different parts of the world, and decided that none of these was perfect. It was also realized that creation of the perfect code, from which unlimited precision and unlimited capacity (i.e. capacity for unlimited expansion for inclusion of new entities without loss of the existing classificatory information) could be demanded, would require several years and should therefore be postponed until the 10th revision. Of the existing codes, we selected the one first introduced by SNOP and further propagated by the American Cancer Society. This is a 3-digit code in which only 8 and 9 are used as first digits, so that the contents are limited to 200 entities. This code has been used extensively and has gained increasing popularity among pathologists. It was created in English but now exists in Japanese. A French and a Portuguese version of the neoplasms section have been published, and a Spanish one is in preparation.

The IARC proposal was presented to the WHO Study Group on Classification of Diseases at its meeting in November 1971. The Group was unable to accept the proposal on the ground that it was not compatible with their earlier decision that only 3 digits should be mandatory for international use. To be meaningful, the system proposed by IARC needed a minimum of 4 digits.

Recognizing that the IARC project had some merit, WHO convened Working Groups to review the proposal and the compromises suggested; these met in March and September 1972.

The Working Groups of WHO proposed that the neoplasms chapter for ICD (9) should comprise the following fields:

Malignant neoplasms	140-199
Neoplasms of lymphatic and hemopoietic tissue	200-209
Benign neoplasms	210-229
Carcinoma in situ	230-234
Other and unspecified neoplasms	235-239

Categories 235 to 238 classify by site certain well-defined tumors whose benign or malignant nature is not certain; category 239 classifies neoplasms for which there is no statement as to whether they are bening or malignant.

The Working Groups recommended that despite several disadvantages, the morphology of neoplasms should be coded internationally according to the scheme used in MOTNAC and that this be incorporated in ICD(9).

ICD (Oncology)

The Working Groups considered that the proposed ICD(9) did not meet the requirements of many workers and endorsed the proposal that there should be a parallel system, compatible with the neoplasms chapter of ICD(9), which would not only permit the coding of morphology for all neoplasms but would also give the same anatomical detail for the benign, in-situ and unspecified cancers as for the malignant ones.

The "behavior" of the neoplasms would be carried in a separate behavior code.
It is thus proposed that WHO issue a separate ICD (Oncology) (ICD(O)) containing the system outlined above. This could also include supplementary classifications considered suitable for international use, e.g. for laterality, staging, etc.

These proposals were accepted at the meeting of the WHO Study Group for the 9th Revision of the ICD held in January 1973 in Geneva.

A few problems remain to be faced - the index, the behavior code, morphological terms for cancer-related conditions, and the extension of the geographical and morphological codes.

Two indexes will be needed, one for ICD(9) and another for ICD(O). These will have to be constructed at the same time to ensure comparability.

Behavior Code

O Benign
1 Uncertain whether benign or malignant
2 Carcinoma in situ
3 Malignant primary site
5 Acute (leukemia)
6 Malignant metastatic
7 Chronic (leukemia)
9 Malignant uncertain whether primary or metastatic site.

The behavior codes used by MOTNAC and SNOP are not identical.

SNOP has two codes:

a) the first is issued with rubrics 800 to 975 of the M code. This consists of O, 1, 2, 3, 6, and 9 of the code above.

b) the second applies to M numbers 980 to 993, i.e. the leukemias. This uses digits 5 and 7 of the code above but 3 now means NOS (no other specification) 8 subacute and 9 a-leukemic.

MOTNAC uses both the behavior codes of SNOP and adds an optional grading code applicable to M numbers 800-975.

Problems that might arise when SNOP and MOTNAC users change to the ICD behavior code must be considered, but the use of a grading code in the same column as the behavior code is not recommended.

Extension of Morphology Code

Coding of a statement according to MOTNAC involves three axes: topography: 4 digits; morphology: 3 digits, behavior: 1 digit.

Topography: The rubrics for topography theoretically provide for 600 terms (140.0 to 199.9). It would be useful to have the code open-ended so that further subdivisions of categories could be produced by those who need them. It would thus be wise to assign five digits for topography.

Morphology: Three digits are used to denote morphology, the first digit being either 8 or 9. This in effect provides for 200 entities, and in MOTNAC/SNOP this is not easily expansible as the next digit is preempted for behavior.

The International Reference Centers for Histopathological Classification of Tumors organized by the Cancer Unit of WHO, Geneva, produce new classifications which are site-specific. Not all the terms utilized can be accommodated within the 200 rubrics.

Certain cancer-related conditions, such as cystic disease of the breast, that should be included in ICD(O) are not within rubrics 800 to 999 of the M code of SNOP. In other than the neoplasms fields of SNOP the M term has 4 digits and the terminal digit has no behavioral significance.

Behavior: The ICD(O) behavior code should not be expanded.

It seems that many of the problems raised above can be solved by setting aside 4 digits for morphology and making separate provision for the behavior code .

Topography (T) Behavior (B) Morphology (M)

Even though the order traditional with SNOP and MOTNAC is topography, morphology, and behavior, it is probably wise to avoid this order since it could lead to confusion about the meaning of the 4th digit of the M term.

Chapter 2 of ICD(9) is divided into 5 sections (malignant, lymphohemopoietic, benign, in situ, unspecified). The ICD(O) behavior code determines to which of these ICD(9) sections an ICD(O) term should be assigned in conversion from ICD(O) to ICD(9). From this point of view, it could be argued that the order should be: behavior, topography, and morphology.

B T M

References

1. International Classification of Diseases, 1965 Revision, Volume I. Geneva: WHO 1967; Volume II. Geneva: WHO 1969.

Histological Classification and its Implications in the Utility of Registry Data in Epidemiological Studies

E. Saxén

The value of cancer registry data in epidemiological studies concerned with cancer is dependent upon the reliability and comparability of the data used. If these data are to be analyzed it is necessary for the material to have been processed with reference to uniform classification and coding systems.To a great extent, progress in science depends upon classification; a given material must be grouped and classified in accordance with fixed criteria if some order is to be obtained from chaos. The classification applied depends on the problem under investigation . However, if a classification system does not lead to logical and useful results it might be wrong, and trials with a new one are required. Currently, the basis of tumor classification is microscopy, which means that a histomorphological classification of tumors is employed.

However, a malignant tumor is a clinical concept - a tumor that will prove fatal if treatment is not given. For decades, the criteria applied by pathologists in the diagnosis of a malignant tumor have developed by means of empirical correlation of the structure of the tumor with the clinical course of the patient. A relatively clear picture of the structural features of fatal tumors has emerged by virtue of retrospective studies.

Consequently, pathologists are now justified in using the originally clinical terms "benign" and "malignant." As a rule, differentiation between a benign and a malignant tumor is not difficult for the pathologist, but the decision made is not absolutely clearcut.

Behavior of tumors is, also the primary axis in their classification according to ICD, i.e. they are classified according to whether they are clinically malignant or benign. Only after this does topography enter the picture, as do other subordinate determinants, such as organotypic classification. This hierarchical order of criteria should be borne in mind, since it often gives rise to confusion and may jeopardize the comparison of data from different sources.

The definition of cancer, i.e. the definition of a malignant tumor is of primary importance to people who make use of cancer registry data, since if the definition of cancer varies in different registries there is no point in comparing their data.

A set of questions was circulated to physicians by the Medical Committee of the Honourable Society for Investigating the Nature and Cure of Cancer in London in 1802, i.e. 170 years ago, with a view to acquiring information on cancer (2).

The first question was: "What are the diagnostic signs of cancer," after this the circular continued "It is very much to be wished that we had an exact definition of cancer, those of the nosologists being very imperfect and insufficient. That we may be able to say something more satisfactory than that it seems to be cancer. It has accordingly happened that a disease which has been denominated cancer by one medical man has not been allowed to be such by another; and painful and hazardous operations have been performed by some, which were not thought necessary, or likely to be successful, by others. Hence an opening has also been made for false pretentions and impositions; and, though no person conversant in practice thinks that a true genuine cancer was ever cured, there is an abundance of cases in which cures of this disease are asserted with the greatest confidence."

During the 16th and 17th centuries, cancer was almost synonymous with a "Verschwärung (fressende, zerstörende Bildung") (destructive growth). As late as in 1855, Virchow stated in his lectures: "Die Mehrzahl der Chirurgen ist noch heutzutage geneigt den Begriff des Krebses nicht zu beschränken auf eine Histologische Form, sondern darunter alles zu verstehen, was bösartig ist" (even now, most surgeons are not inclined to restrict the concept of cancer to a particular histological form; they apply the term to any malignant growth) (17).Those of us working in cancer registries are bound to ask ourselves whether the situation is much better now than it was 170 years ago,when the Committee wrote: "It is much to be wished that we may no longer be deceived by ambiguous words and phrases, or consider them as conveying to us any essential or practical knowledge."

At present the best classification seems to be a histological one. As was pointed out above, this does not represent a clearcut decision, but an interpretation of tissue changes by an individual pathologist. Pathologists provide information that is of crucial importance in the diagnosis of tumors and treatment of patients, but it should be remembered that the human observer is the least standardized of all sources of data analyzed in medicine. The observer variability may thus be considerable, and consequently data from different areas may not be mutually comparable. Diagnosis on the basis of morphology is subject to definite limitations.

One of these limitations is illustrated by the preinvasive and so-called carcinoma-in-situ lesions. Nowadays, it is a common practice to apply the same cytomorphological criteria of malignancy to lesions detected by microscopy in clinically healthy people as are applied to clinically diagnosed tumors. It has not yet been proved whether this is justified, although some statistical and certain experimental data (13) point in this direction. In areas in which all these lesions are registered as malignant tumors and treated as such, the observed incidence of tumors at a given site is bound to increase, and an improvement is inevitably noted in the survival statistics. It is not known whether this results from effective treatment, early diagnosis, or the possibility that benign lesions are also treated as malignant. A man-made epidemic of carcinoma in situ of the uterine cervix in Finland is illustrated in Fig. 1, which shows the tremendous increase in carcinoma-in-situ lesions when mass examinations are started and this diagnosis applied. Another example within the same area is microinvasive carcinoma of the cervical canal. If cases of carcinoma in situ with "buds" and early invasive "occult" carcinomas are grouped under this joint heading, a definite improvement of the therapeutic results will ensue, since apparently the former does not differ in clinical behavior from the usual carcinoma-in-situ lesion.

The "incidence" and prevalence of these lesions depends not only upon their definition, but also upon the magnitude of the mass screening program, and the age groups screened.

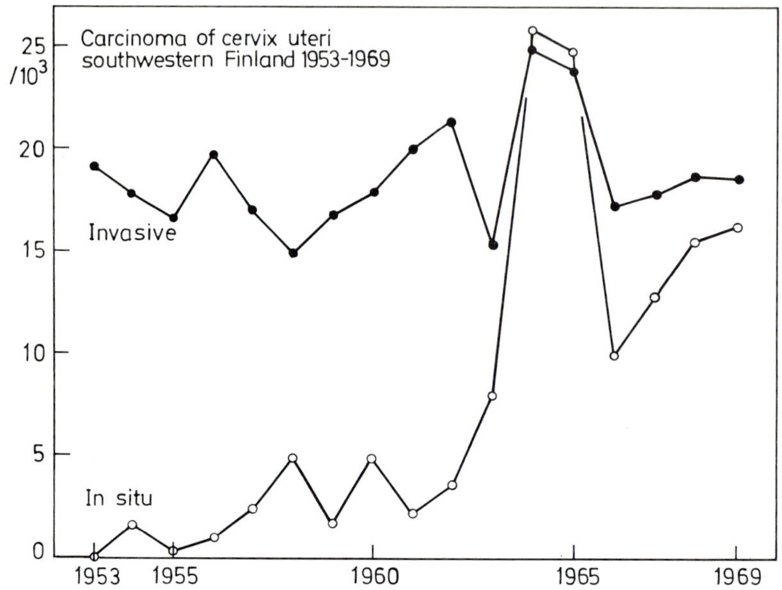

Finnish
cancer registry

Fig. 1. Incidence of cervical cancer and of reported Ca-in-situ lesions in Finland, 1960-1968

Another and somewhat different example of the difficulties experienced in the definition of malignancy is provided by latent carcinoma of the prostate in elderly men. There is wide discrepancy in the observed occurrence of latent and clinically manifest carcinoma of the prostate. Many autopsy studies made in different countries have indicated a high frequency (25-34%) of prostatic carcinoma in series of men of over 40 years of age. Fig. 2 is from a recent study in Norway, illustrating the situation there (10). The "incidence" of this type of cancer depends upon the frequency of autopsies and upon the care with which autopsies are performed.

Furthermore, it is well known that it is almost impossible to compare the incidence figures of transitional cell neoplasms of the urinary bladder in different areas. The distinction between papillomas and papillomatous carcinomas varies, and the terminology applied is often a confusing mixture of cytological and histopathological classifications

The over-diagnosis of thyroid malignancies provides a further example of the lack of uniform definition of malignancy and of observer variability. On re-examination of 38 so-called "malignant adenomas" reported to the Finnish Cancer Registry, it was found that 60 percent of them (23 cases) were benign tumors - a finding that was also confirmed by a ten-year follow-up of the patients (15). Similar over-diagnosing may occur in the case of melanomas in children, as has been demonstrated (14).

The value of organotypic classification of cancer in the provision of more exact and more reliable data is indisputable. However, it should be used together with topography. Distribution by histological type alone does not give much useful information, as illustrated by a table extracted from one cancer register recording the distribution of histological types according to the SNOP classification (Table 1).

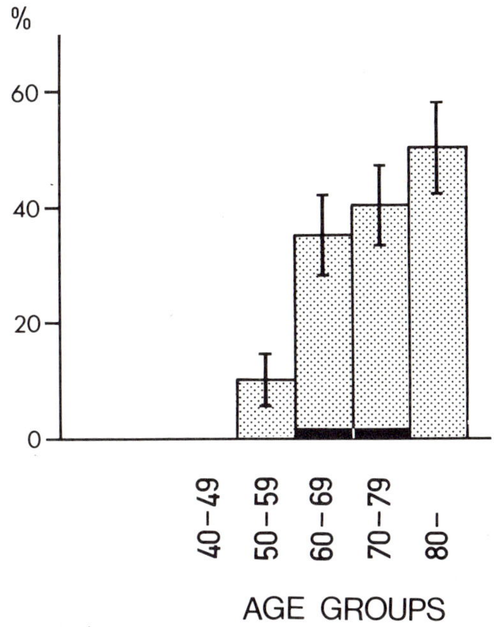

Fig. 2 Prevalence of prostatic cancer in 206 consecutive autopsies in Oslo, Norway (from HARBITZ and HAUGER, 1972)

Table 1. Distribution by histological type of tumors of the ten most frequent cancer sites

	Men (%)	Women (%)
Squamous cell carcinomas	32.7	24.2
Adenocarcinomas	24.9	17.9
Basal cell carcinomas	17.5	15.7

Of the tumors of the ten most frequent cancer sites in men, 32.7 percent were squamous cell carcinomas, 24.9 percent adenocarcinomas, and 17.5 percent basal cell carcinomas, whereas in women 24.2 percent were squamous cell carcinomas, 17.9 percent adenocarcinomas, and 15.7 percent basal cell carcinomas. Some doubt is attached to the utility of information of this nature.

A real difficulty with histological classification arises when multiple axes are used in the classification of tumors, i.e. a topographical classification for some tumors, a morphological one for some others, and perhaps a biochemical or etiological classification for others. Tumors of the lymphatic and hematopoietic tissues provide an example of this.

The epidemiology of cancer of the nasopharynx is appreciably different from that of nasopharyngeal carcinoma. In the former situation, but not in the latter, lymphomas may or may not be included in the material, and depending upon the area concerned, this could account for from 1 percent of the cases in Taiwan (19) to 29 percent in Denmark (11).

Even more confusion could arise from the diagnosis lymphoepithelioma, which is now regarded as a form of squamous cell carcinoma but still referred to as a malignant lymphoma in some studies. The percentage of this type of tumor varies from 3 in Taiwan (19) to 32 in Bombay (16). If no histological examination is performed all lymphomas are classified as nasopharyngeal cancer; if a histological examination is performed, up to 30 percent of lymphomas may be transferred to the category of tumors of the lymphatic tissue in some areas.

The situation is very similar with tumors of the small intestine. In Iran, 90 percent of malignant tumors of the small intestine are lymphosarcomas according to BAREKET et al. (1); according to VUORI (18), the corresponding percentage in Finland is 18 (Table 2).

Table 2. Frequency of lymphomas and other malignant tumors of the small intestine in Iran and Finland

Iran	(BAREKET et al.)	1962-1969	lymphomas	= 64 cases
			other types of cancer	= 6 cases
Finland	(VUORI)	1953-1962	lymphomas	= 32 cases
			other types of cancer	= 148 cases

In both series, the percentage of histological confirmation is high. From this it follows that if the malignant lymphomas are grouped as tumors of the lymphatic tissues, and not with reference to the primary site, i.e. the small intestine, malignant tumors of the small intestine are rare in Iran but more common in Finland. However, if the percentage of histological confirmation had been very low, the malignant lymphomas would have been grouped as tumors of the small intestine, and the incidence of these tumors might perhaps be the same in both countries. Fig. 3 illustrates the variation in site distribution of the different tumors.

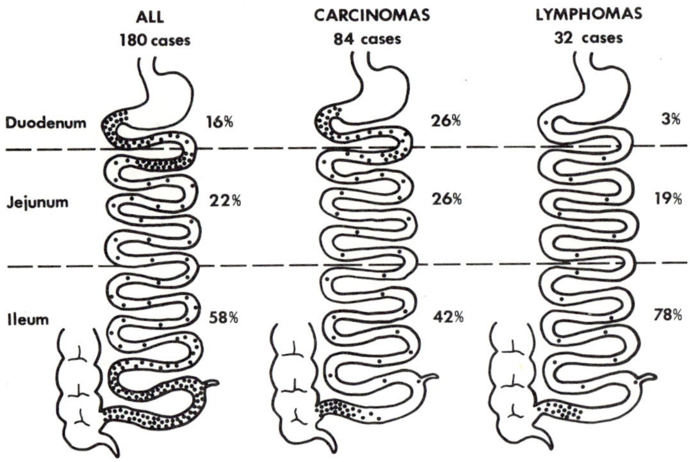

Fig. 3. Site distribution of carcinomas and lymphomas of the small intestine in Finland (18)

These two examples, tumors of the nasopharynx and tumors of the small intestine, demonstrate the danger inherent in the independent use of multiple axes, in this case topography and morphology.

A great deal of information is obviously lost if all the malignant tumors of a single organ are assigned to one group. The special characteristics of one type of cancer (e.g. lymphomas) may be hidden under the features of other types. This clearly proves the value of histological classification. Consequently, the specific histological types of one organ should be studied separately, and also epidemiologically, instead of all cancers being grouped together. The value of this approach has been illustrated in earlier studies (15) as far as thyroid cancer is concerned. The relative survival curves for three different histological types of thyroid carcinoma are indicated in Fig.4,

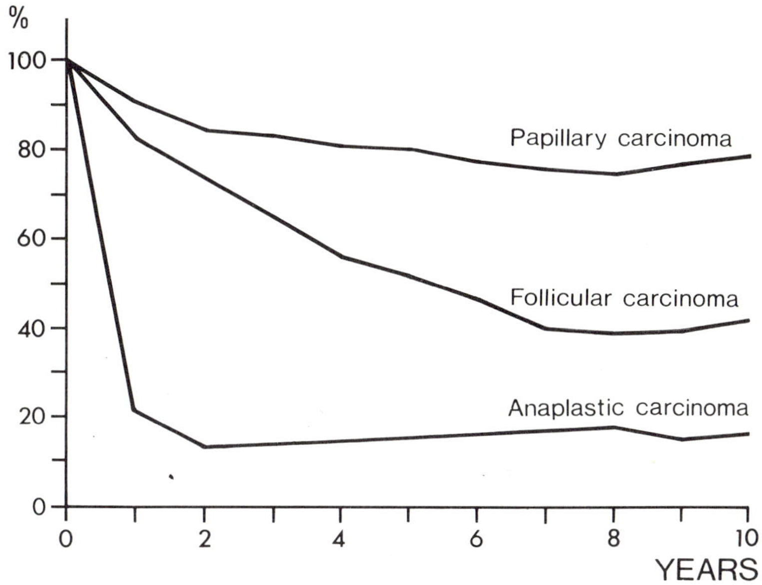

Relative survival curves for three different histological types of thyroid carcinoma in Finland 1958-1962 (7)

and the frequency of inoperable tumors and the occurence of metastases classified by histological type in Table 3 (7). The major biological differences in the various histological types are clearly seen. Cancer registry material is not as yet suitable for this kind of study, as it is usually based upon diagnoses made by many pathologists applying different criteria (Table 4). If histological diagnoses are to be made as comparable as possible, a uniformly accepted classification is required. At the moment, comparable results are practicable only if the same pathologist examines all the slides of the total material to be compared. This observer variability has also been shown in the case of lung cancer (5, 11), in cancer of the female breast (3), and in malignant lymphomas (9). The occurrence of these inconsistencies must be borne in mind in comparison of statistical analyses.

The value of histological classification is also seen when skin tumors are discussed.

Table 3. Frequency of inoperable tumors and metastases by histological type of thyroid carcinomas diagnosed in Finland, 1958-1962 (Franssila 1971)

	No. of cases	Inoperable tumors (%)	Metastases Regional (%)	Distant (%)
Papillary carcinoma	100	8	42	13
Follicular carcinoma	60	6	2	70
Medullary carcinoma	10	-	70	10
Anaplastic carcinoma	58	47	28	45
Others	3	-	33	67
All cases	231	17	29	36

Table 4. Correlation of the diagnoses of thyroid cancer in the original Finnish Cancer Registry material in 1958-1962 and the re-examined material (8)

Cancer registry material	Re-examined material			
	Total	Anapl. ca. 1	Follic. ca. 2	Papill. ca. 3
Total	345	63	48	96
Anapl. ca.	67	47	6	--
Follic. ca.	53	1	15	13
Papill. ca.	64	2	1	53

Table 5. Tumors of the skin in Finland, 1969. Distribution by site and histology (Finnish Cancer Registry)

	Total	Basal cell carcinomas	Squamous cell carcinomas	Melanomas
Face and neck	1177	1012	120	36
Trunk	178	93	13	61
Extremities	129	42	24	57
	1484	1147	157	154

Table 5 lists the frequency of different forms of malignant skin tumors by site in Finland in 1969. Of the tumors in the face and neck, 75 percent are basaliomas, but the corresponding percentage in the extremities is no more than 17. This indicates the necessity of knowing whether basal cell carcinomas are included in the cancer registry data or not.

If satisfactory results are to be obtained, detailed topographical classification must be supplemented by histological classification. The WHO program for histopathological definition and classification of tumors might prove of value in this respect. However, it should be remembered that other, and perhaps more useful classifications may become available in the near future. For lymphomas, mention may be made of the origin of lymphocytes and the specific products of lymphocytes, and for some other tumors the etiology and antigenic relationships as revealed by cytotoxicity tests.

It is well known from experimental pathology that neoplasms that are different in morphology can be identical in etiology (Polyoma virus). Accordingly, we should perhaps not be too concerned with morphological classifications alone. Morphological studies, important as they are, present only one fact of the classification of tumors, and information may thus be lost if tumors of different morphology are too sharply separated.

Furthermore, it could also be emphasized that the situation is made even more confusing by the fact that the "organ" frequently employed as the basis in topographic classification is not necessarily a useful entity. Not only may various components of the "organ" be derived from very different embryonic cell populations; tissue components with close morphological similarities in the same organ may also have had a different developmental history. One example of this is the mucosa of the urinary bladder, in which the trigonum is developmentally very different from the rest of the bladder. It is thus conceivable that these cells also possess different potencies as far as malignant transformation is concerned.

Another developmentally misleading concept is the "epithelium," and the malignant tumor, carcinoma, derived from epithelial cells. Epithelial structures in the organism have derived from all the embryonic layers; as a consequence, tumors that are morphologically classifiable as carcinomas may have an ectodermal (skin), entodermal (liver) or mesodermal (kidney) origin. To take the matter one step further, even a typical epidermoid carcinoma may have these very different developmental backgrounds: cf. epidermoid carcinoma of the skin (ectoderm), of the lung (entoderm), and of the pelvis (mesoderm).

Summary and Conclusions

The basis of present-day tumor classification is microscopy. However, histological classification cannot be independent of site classification. The best results seem to be achieved with a detailed topographical classification of malignant tumors supplemented by a histological classification in accordance with strict and well-defined criteria. A great deal of information is lost if malignant tumors of one specific site are treated as a single group in epidemiological studies. In general, cancer registry material is not yet suitable for comparative studies of different histological types of tumors, as it is based upon diagnoses made by pathologists applying different criteria. The development of opportunities for the employment of a classification based upon methods resulting from basic research should be followed carefully; this would not only permit of easier measurement but would also be less subjective in nature.

References

1. BAREKAT, A. A., SAIDI, F., DUTZ, W.: Cancer survey in south Iran with special reference to gastrointestinal neoplasms. Int. J. Cancer 7, 353 (1971).
2. Cancer Problems 160 years ago. Int. J. Cancer 2, 281 (1967).
3. CUTLER, S. J., BLACK, M. M., FRIEDELL, G. H., VIDONE,R. A., GOLDENBERG, I. S.: Prognostic factors in cancer of the female breast. II. Reproducibility of histopathologic classification. Cancer 19, 75 (1966).
4. FAULKNER, J. W., DOCKERTY, M. E.: Lymphosarcoma of the small intestine. Surg Gynec. Obstet. 95, 76 (1952).
5. FEINSTEIN, A. R., GOLFMAN, N. A., YESNER, R.: Observer variability in the histopathologic diagnosis of lung cancer. Ann. Rev. resp. Dis. 101, 671 (1970).
6. Finnish Cancer Registry: Cancer Incidence in Finland 1969. Helsinki:Cancer Society of Finland (publ. no. 18) 1972.
7. FRANSSILA, K.: Value of histologic classification of thyroid cancer. Acta path. microbiol. scand. Suppl. 225 (1971).
8. FRANSSILA, K., SAXÉN, E.: Histologic classification as a problem in the epidemiology of thyroid cancer. In: Recent Results in Cancer Research. Vol. 39. Ed. E. Grundmann, H. Tulinius, Berlin-Heidelberg-New York: Springer 1972.
9. HAKAMA, M., FRANSSILA, K., SAXÉN, E.: Reliability of frequency figures for malignant lymphomas. Ann. clin. Res. 1973. In press.
10. HARBITZ, T. B., HAUGEN, O. A.: Histology of the prostate in elderly men. Acta path. microbiol. scand. A 80, 756 (1972).
11. LARSSON, S.: Completeness and reliability of lung cancer registration in the Swedish Cancer Registry. Acta path. microbiol. scand. A 79, 389 (1971).
12. MUIR, C. S.: Nasopharyngeal carcinoma in non-Chinese populations with special reference to South-east Asia and Africa. Int. J. Cancer 8, 351 (1971).
13. SAKSELA, E., MEYER, B.: Cell-mediated cytoxicity against HeLa cells in patients with invasive and preinvasive cervical cancer. J. nat. Cancer Institute 1973. In press.
14. SAKSELA, E., RINTALA, A.: Misdiagnosis of prepubertal malignant melanoma. Reclassification of a cancer registry material. Cancer 22, 1308 (1968).
15. SAXÉN, E., FRANSSILA, K., HAKAMA, M.: Effect of histological typing of registry material on the results of epidemiological comparison in thyroid cancer. In: Thyroid Cancer. UICC Monograph Series Vol. 12. Ed. C. Hedinger, p.98. Berlin-Heidelberg-New York: Springer 1970.
16. WAHI, P. N.: Malignant tumors of the nasopharynx and accessory sinuses in India. In: Cancer of the Nasopharynx. UICC Monograph Series Vol. 1, p.24. Copenhagen: Munksgaard 1967.
17. VIRCHOW, R.: Die Vorlesungen Rudolf Virchows über Allgemeine Pathologische Anatomie. Ed. E. Kugler. Jena: Gustav Fischer 1930.
18. VUORI, J.: Primary malignant tumors of the small intestine diagnosed in Finland 1953-1962 (in Finnish). Thesis, University of Turku 1970.
19. YEH, S.: Histology of nasopharyngeal cancer. In: Cancer of the Nasopharynx. UICC Monograph Series Vol. 1, p. 147. Copenhagen: Munksgaard 1967.

Uses of Cancer Registry Data for Planning and Administration of a Cancer Control Program

I. Martinez

This paper reviews the uses of Cancer Registry data already published and their potential uses in the computer age.

The presentation is based on data derived from a population-based cancer registry with follow-up of the patients.

Cancer makes up a group of diseases which should be under a governmentally controlled program. It is accepted that a cancer control program is a coordinated group of administrative, professional and technical activities directed toward the prevention, detection, and diagnosis of cancer and the treatment and rehabilitation of patients with the disease. Moreover, the program should include clinical, epidemiological, and experimental research directed at the improvement of current knowledge and management of the disease. The participation of not only clinician and pathologist but in addition of epidemiologist, statistician, health educator, visiting nurse, social worker, therapist, health administrator, and computer programmer is vital to a program of this kind.

A cancer control program can become a complex and rather expensive enterprise. No matter what its size or coverage, it needs the best use of the resources available. To this end it is necessary to plan carefully, monitor activities within the program, evaluate the results of treatment. Data on the distribution of cancer in the community are indispensable, as are data on the demographic, cultural, and economic composition of the population and data relative to the professional and physical resources available in the community where cancer cases are diagnosed.

The data about cancer in a community can be obtained from other different sources, e.g. mortality data, survey data. However, there is general agreement that the best source of data is a well-organized, well-managed population-based cancer registry with follow-up of the patients.
Such a cancer registry in the planning and administration of a cancer control program can have various practical uses. Its records show, for example, the Total Number of New and Active Cancer Cases and Total Number of Deaths. This crude information gives us an idea of the numerical size of the problem, especially when it is compared with corresponding information on other diseases in the community. With these data we can begin to estimate the overall resources necessary to comply with the objectives of the cancer control program. The periodic changes in these crude figures are used to modify the program accordingly.

Distributions of Cases, Deaths, and Rates by Primary Site, Sex, and Age are also recorded by cancer registries. These distributions allow more specific planning and ordering of priorities. Obviously, a program to control cancer of the cervix uteri will be planned and administered differently in Israel than in Connecticut, Puerto Rico, or Colombia. In any program the sexes and different age groups (children, adults of reproductive age, aging adults, etc.) must be arranged in order of priority.

A good administrator will be careful to make the necessary adjustments when the disease or population patterns change. It is important to budget according to the more efficient aspect of the cancer control activities, following modern public health concepts.

It is useful to consult the distributions of Cases and Rates by Primary Sites and Socioeconomic Status Including Occupation of the Patients as the known different frequencies of some cancer sites at different social levels and in some occupations lead us to plan quite different control programs for the various social classes in the community. These distributions are particularly useful in planning research studies. The administration will be somewhat difficult when the lowest social strata are disproportionately highly represented in the community. In such situations greater variety in resources will be needed.

The administration of a control program for cancer of the stomach in Japan is quite different than a similar activity in Chile or Iceland. In general, the pattern of cancer sites and resources distribution are different in highly industrialized communities than in underdeveloped ones.

Distributions of Cases and Rates by Primary Site and Residence of the Patients have been used to plan many epidemiological studies searching for environmental factors associated with the disease. The residence of the patients, however, will determine the distribution of the resources in a good proportion of cases.

If the patient with cancer, or the apparently healthy person, must travel long distances to get services, the probabilities of delay and defaulting are higher.

The administration will consider the convenience of costs and productivity of the different available alternatives. Preventive or corrective measures recommended by the research studies should be put into practice.

Cases and Percentages are also classified by Primary Site and by Method and Place of Diagnosis. The finding of high percentages of (a) cases without histological diagnosis, (b) incomplete or incorrect medical records, and (c) patients with cancer at certain primary sites who have not been discussed at tumor clinics or tumor boards means that it is necessary to plan a professional education program or the redistribution of resources, or both.

The evolution of these indices will be used by the administration to evaluate, at least in part, the quality of diagnosis of cancer in the community and institutions.

It is accepted in general that the earlier the stage of the disease at diagnosis the higher the patient's chances of survival are, other conditions being equal.
The finding of high percentages of cases not diagnosed until the advanced stages and of long intervals between the first symptoms and the date of diagnosis indicate the need for a study to explain this situation. The most frequent conditions associated with high percentages of these indices are lack of basic knowledge of the disease and of the location and use of resources available among the public, lack of

professional and physical resources, indifference and lack of understanding of the disease among physicians, and absence of cancer detection programs. These deficiencies are usually all present in varying degrees of intensity, and frequently a mixed type of corrective program is needed. Indices by primary site and interval between first symptoms and diagnosis are useful in the evaluation of the effectiveness of the established programs, including the cancer detection programs, of the community. Sometimes the presentation of these indices compared with those of other areas have been enough to prove doctors' attitudes. It is necessary to know how many malignant tumors have been observed of what type, and at what stage the malignant tumors did not receive conventional treatment. It is also important to know the survival rates of the treated patients classified by site, stage and type of treatment, and how the survival rate compares with that in other areas. Significantly low survival rates merit detailed studies in order to find the causes and indicate the measures necessary to improve them. Sometimes the finding of differences in survival of patients with different types of treatment in the same area leads to detailed and properly designed clinical trials.

In this computer era, the Cancer Registry is able to provide each physician and hospital with a feedback of the pertinent information on patients they are treating, their survival, and results in other areas or institutions for comparison. It is a simple mechanism of auto-evaluation. Observation of the trends in these indices over the years is very useful in evaluation of the programs of professional education, availability of resources, and to a certain extent the degree of public education.

When a high percentage of tumors are treated by radical surgery of certain organs, a plan of physical and emotional rehabilitation must be initiated. These distribution data are used administratively to justify the quest for resources to support the corrective program.

Findings of Significant Variation of Time Trends in Cancer Incidence and Differences between Groups, Areas, and Countries have been the most frequent source of epidemiological studies in both the domestic and the international fields. In spite of the incomplete uniformity of methods of diagnosis, classification, registry and treatment of lesions, the material from cancer registries are of a caliber to permit discovery of etiological clues. They are making significant contributions to knowledge of the disease, as is frequently seen in the literature. There are various ways in which the registry material is useful for these purposes: some physical, social, and cultural information previously collected by the registry about the patient is available; study cases are already available or arrive systematically, and sampling of these cases is easy; the registry also provides useful control groups.

Computerization of the Registry permits quicker retrieval of data by small groups or areas affected, which means they can be linked with factors thought to be associated. A surveillance program of this type may constitute the beginning of a detailed investigation which allows discovery of some etiological clues. Trends in cancer incidence rates classified by age and primary sites can also be used in formulations of predictions of the future incidence of cancer. This forecasting should form the basis of a largescale plan for a national cancer control program.

Many aspects of cancer are not yet known in all areas of the disease. The best diagnosis and treatment of certain types of tumors require highly trained professional personnel and very expensive equipment. Talent for research is not very abundant. For these reasons, incorporation of these resources into the so-called cancer research centers has been considered. The data stored by a Cancer Registry is indispensable in planning such cancer research centers. Failure to use these data will jeopardize the future success of such centers. It is therefore logical that a cancer registry should be one of the operational units of this type of center, increasing and detailing the information input from the clinical records. One aspect of good administration is the provision of adequate training for personnel. Cancer registry data is essential to both in-service and academic training of medical and paramedical personnel.

References

1. ACHESON, R. M., BAILAR, J. C., CORREA, P., CUTLER, S.J., GAITAN, M. MARTÎNEZ, I., RINGEL, A., ZIPPIN, C.: Seminar on Cancer Registries in Latin America. Pan-American Health Organization, WHO, 1970. English translation of "Seminarios sobre Registros de Câncer en América Latina", PAHO, WHO. Pub.científica No. 215, 1970.
2. BLUM, H. L., KERANEN, G. M.: Control of Chronic Diseases in Man. New York: Am. Pub. Hlth. Ass. 1966.
3. BRESLOW, L.: Cancer. Vol. 6. Chap. 21. The Prevention of Cancer. Ed. R. W. Raven. London: Butterworth 1959.
4. DAVIES, J. M.: Searching for Occupational Cancer Risks. Trans. Soc. occup. Med. 18, 42 (1968).
5. DOLL, R., PAYNE, P., WATERHOUSE, J.: Cancer Incidence in Five Continents. UICC. Vol. 1, 1966, Vol. 2, 1970. Berlin-Heidelberg-New York: Springer.
6. EVANG, K., PEDERSEN, E.: Public Health Aspects of Cancer Control. J. chron. Dis. 11, 149 (1960).
7. LILIENFELD, A. M., PEDERSEN, E., DOWD, J. E.: Cancer Epidemiology: Methods of Study. Baltimore: Johns Hopkins Univ. Press 1967.
8. GROHAM, W.: Disease Control Programs. Cancer. Program Analysis. Washington, D. C.: U. S. Dept. H. E. W. 1966.
9. HAENZEL, W., LOURIE, W. I.: Quality Control Data in a large-scale Cancer Registry Program. Methods of Information in Medicine, 5, 2, 67-74 (1966).
10. HAENZEL, W. et al.: Statistical approaches to the Study of Cancer with particular reference to Cancer Registries. J. chron. Dis. 4, 589 (1956).
11. International Agency for Research on Cancer: Report of the Meeting on Sources of Cancer Statistics. Lyon, Nov., 1968.
12. MARTINEZ, I., ED.: Cancer in Puerto Rico, 1950-1964, 1965-1970. Cancer Control Program. Puerto Rico: Department of Health, Santurce.
13. PAYNE, P. M.: The Principles of Cancer Registration. In: Cancer Vol. 6, Chap. 19. Ed. Raven, R. W. London: Butterworth 1959.
14. PEDERSEN, E.: Some Uses of the Cancer Registry in Cancer Control. Brit. J. prev. Med. 16, 105 (1962).
15. STOCKS, P.: Cancer Registration and Studies of Incidence by Surveys. Bull. WHO, 20, 697 (1959).
16. TEPPO, L., HAKOLINEN, T., SAFEN, E.: The Prediction of Cancer Incidence in Finland for the Year 1980, by means of Cancer Registry Material. To be published in Int. J. Epidemiology.
17. WHO: Early Detection of Cancer. Tech. Rep. Series No. 422. Geneva: 1969.
18. WHO, IARC, DOLL, R.: Incidence Data Currently Available and their use. Meeting on Sources of Cancer Statistics, Nov., 1968.

19. WHO: Prevention of Cancer. Tech. Rep. Series No. 276. Geneva 1964.
20. WHO: Cancer Control. Tech. Rep. Series No. 251. Geneva 1963.
21. WHO: Experts Committee on Health Statistics, (Fifth Report). Tech. Rep. Series No. 133, 1957.
22. WHO: Experts Committee on Health Statistics, (Second Report). Tech. Rep. Series No. 25, 1950.
23. WAKEFIELD, J., et al.: Public Education about Cancer. Cancer Education Programmes in Various Countries. A Tech. Rep. Geneva: UICC. 1967.
24. WECKWORTH, V. E.: Development and Use of Registries. Proceedings of the Institute on "Development of Community Health Services for Congenital Abnormities. Ann Arbor: Michigan University Press 1963.

The United States Network of Cancer Registries

W. Haenszel

Sources of U. S. Data on Cancer Incidence and Patient Survival

The consensus of cancer registry experts is that there is an upper limit possibly in the order of 4-5,000,000, to the size of a population that can be effectively monitored by a single registry. A larger population base multiplies the number of hospitals and physicians the registry staff deals with, with the result that the system becomes less responsive and the timely exchange of information between registry and reporting sources is impeded. A national registry is well suited to countries of the size of Denmark, but for larger countries the solution lies in a decentralized network of cancer registries. One prototype for decentralization is provided by England and Wales, where cancer registries are administered by the Regional Hospital Boards and the Registrar-Generals's office has the responsibility for collation of the data from regional registries for national reports (1).

Up to 1970 little serious thought had been given in the United States to the systematic development of a network of registries or to specification of the characteristics of such a system and of the objectives to be served. This was due in part to the fact that the National Cancer Institute had two separate, functioning methods for the collection of data on incidence and end-results. Incidence data on a national scale have been assembled by ad hoc morbidity surveys; the first such survey was conducted in 1937-39, the second in 1947-48, and the third, now nearing completion, covers the years 1969-71 (2). The current morbidity survey is more elaborate than its predecessors and has included interviews with samples of patients for information on site-specific etiologic factors and on treatment costs. The Biometry Branch of the National Cancer Institute has relied on complex computer procedures for editing and processing the returns from the field offices covering two States and seven metropolitan areas. One drawback of the morbidity survey technique is the time required for planning and clearances with interested parties in local communities. It was decided in advance that the Third National Cancer Survey would be the last of its kind in the United States. This decision also recognized that while morbidity surveys can produce good quality incidence data, a continuing registry operation is obviously superior for studies of end results.

The source of patient survival data has been a group of hospital and population-based registries, known as the End Results Group, organized soon after the 1956 National Cancer Conference. The composition of members reflected a response to an immediate need by registries in a position to supply data, rather than deliberate design. Nevertheless, the series of reports published by the End Results Group have provided valuable descriptive data on patient survival experience in the United States (3). The program has also served as a pilot and testing ground for development of the reporting and management techniques necessary for the operation of a decentralized network of registries (4).

These arrangements have been made obsolete by the advent of the National Cancer Program, the implementation of which will require information to be supplied by cancer registries for administrative purposes. An enlarged role for population-based registries as sources of data on both cancer incidence and therapeutic end results was obviously indicated. However, wihtin these broadly defined goals there has been no consensus of opinion on the scope and composition of a registry network. Advocates could be found for a wide variety of options, ranging from establishment of cancer registries in each State to assist physicians and hospitals in the follow-up and management of their cancer patients and to assemble information needed for the design of treatment facilities, to the other extreme of designating a limited, carefully selected set of registries, adequately staffed by clinicians, epidemiologists and statisticians, who could study in depth problems pinpointed by the registry data. The latter concept emphasizes the cancer registry as a research tool and resource.

To resolve the complex issues and to formulate an appropriate strategy, in 1971 the National Cancer Institute's Division of Cancer Cause and Prevention appointed an Advisory Committee on Population-based Epidemiology Research Centers, with broad representation of institutional and specialty interests. While one cannot expect that the Committee's recommendations will be followed in every detail, its thorough, dispassionate review has provided a blueprint for a comprehensive, well-rounded cancer registry system for the United States and a set of guidelines for implementation by NCI staff. A summary of the Committee's major findings follows:

1) NCI should develop a coordinated program of cancer surveillance, descriptive epidemiology and end results evaluation. The output of this multi-purpose program should be the basis for:
   a) prompt identification of secular trends in specific cancers;
   b) identification of variations in disease incidence that may lead to etiological hypotheses;
   c) assessment of the efficiency and quality of the medical care system;
   d) studies by which primary and secondary preventive measures can be evaluated.

2) Localities participating in the Third National Cancer Survey should be evaluated as potential candidates for the expanded registry network because they have professional and technical personnel trained in relevant methodology, and also because of their established rapport with the medical community, without which no registry can succeed. Recruitment of additional participants should not, however, be limited to this group.

3) The findings from the Third National Cancer Survey should be used to identify those registries and populations offering the greatest and most immediate study potential.

4) The descriptive incidence data from population-based registries should lay the groundwork for investigations focused on etiology, in the form of either analytic epidemiological studies or animal experiments.

5) The existing End Results Group should constitute the nucleus for an expanded data base on patient survival experience. The Group has a special role to play in the evaluation of long-term results of treatment.

6) The objectives enumerated require an optimum mixture of participating registries, with representation from the following sources:
   a) Individual hospitals specializing in cancer (e.g. Memorial Hospital, New York City) and other university-affiliated treatment centers. Such institutions can provide accurate and specific diagnostic and therapeutic information, high-quality data on patients with relatively rare tumors, access to high-risk patients with potentially precancerous conditions and/or atypical findings in routine screening tests.
   b) Comprehensive Cancer Research Centers, which may be loosely defined as hospitals specializing in cancer, augmented by special research facilities (examples: M. D. Anderson Hospital, Houston; Roswell Park Memorial Institue, Buffalo). These centers provide the milieu for interdisciplinary research and training which are fundamental to advances in cancer control.
   c) Population-based cancer registries. These will provide the bulk of the descriptive data on incidence and endresults.
   d) Population-Based Cancer Study Centers. In addition to maintaining surveillance and reporting in incidence and end results, these centers will conduct epidemiological and clinically oriented studies. They will augment the conventional registry effort with diagnostic, therapeutic, epidemilogic, statistical, laboratory, and other skills on which valid data on incidence and end results depend. Some of the Centers may be part of a Comprehensive Cancer Research Center; others may be closely allied with strong departments of medicine, surgery, and pathology with special interests in cancer. The Population-Based Study Centers will enhance the opportunities for controlled clinical trials among truly representative samples of cases.

7) NCI research and program goals do not presently require, or even suggest an ultimate need for, the establishment of a large-scale national program of cancer registration.

The two levels of effort proposed by the Committee represented in the hierarchical relationships--(1) population-based registries/population-based cancer study centers, and (2) cancer specialty hospitals/comprehensive cancer research centers--deserve special comment. This was the Committee's solution for meeting the competing requirements for representative coverage of a broad population spectrum and for intensive studies in favorable research settings. This compromise proposes deployment of the resources among data collection, data analysis and support of special studies in a manner that could maximize the information obtained while recognizing that personnel and financial resources are finite. While optimum allocations remain a question for reasoned debate, the dangers of extreme maldistributions of effort are obvious. To allocate all the resources to data collection at the expense of no pay-off in information from data analysis would clearly be unprofitable. The other extreme of highly sophisticated studies concentrated in very few localities would also be dangerous, since they would depend on extrapolations from a limited base in the absence of data on representative national experience.

While the Committee guidelines provide the conceptual framework for a network of multi-purpose tumor registries, implementation will require resolution of several issues including: criteria for inclusion of participants, funding, and provisions for national coordination of the registry network.

Selection of Registries. When considered in the abstract, the selection of individual registries poses hard choices. The problem does not lie in the assessment of the strength and weaknesses of any individual registry; these can be recognized. The more difficult problem is the evaluation of the potential contributions of two or more individual registries in relation to the desired characteristics of the larger registry network. In the latter setting one rarely finds clear-cut choices. The network must, of course, be developed with due consideration of the distribution of participating registries by region of the country, characteristics of the population covered (race , ethnic group, urban and rural residence, occupational and other environmental exposures, presence of unique study facilities), and appropriate level of activity (registry or study center).

However, the problems of implementation may not be as formidable as they appear at first glance, since there will be no immediate confrontation by irrevocable choices. Perhaps the most interesting conclusion of the Advisory Committee was that the issue of the initial scope of the registry network is a moot point. Relatively few localities have the necessary program resources and there exists a severe shortage of experienced staff capable of developing and/or operating population-based registries. The immediate decisions will reduce to the designation of a few, strategically placed centers. Expansion of the network must then proceed slowly over a period of years in phase with an enlarging pool of manpower and development of new registry capacities. Options for expansion can be exercised sequentially in the light of experience and new additions judged on an appraisal of the cost-benefit ratios of their potential contributions. These decisions should not be made solely by NCI staff, and a review mechanism must be established that will give due weight to the views of outside consultants.

The existing shortage of trained personnel makes it vital that population-based cancer study centers be utilized for the training of epidemiologists, statisticians, and allied personnel. The importance of training facilities as a criterion for the designation of population-based study centers cannot be overemphasized.

Funding. Individual registries have been financed from a variety of sources. Virtually all the individual hospital and population-based registries were initiated with local sources of funding. The registries which joined the End Results Group received supplements from the National Cancer Institute, which did not replace local funds but were intended to cover the increased costs incurred by membership in the End Results Group. However, in recent years the NCI has assumed an increasing proportion of the costs of supporting population-based cancer registries, and it is reasonable to assume that this trend will continue. One of the major constraints on the size of the registry network envisaged will be the amount of direct or indirect support that NCI will be able to channel to individual registries (or study centers). The question of NCI funding is complex and not easy to discuss due to the multiple sources of funding within NCI. The Institute is not a monolithic organization and the extent of decentralization of review and decision on applications for grant and contract support is not always fully appreciated. Given the multiple objectives to be served by the registry network it seems inevitable that they must rely on multiple sources of funding from NCI. The current policy is best summarized by the guidelines for support of cancer reporting systems and tumor registries approved by the Director of NCI in September 1972.

a) Hospital tumor registries whose primary purpose is to promote continuity of medical follow-up of individual patients should be supported by agencies and programs concerned with the delivery of medical care rather than by NCI.
b) Comprehensive cancer research centers should have tumor registries to describe the patient populations they serve and to evaluate the results of therapy. Such registries should be an integral part of the center's program and should be supported by the NCI Center Grants Program.
c) A network of reporting systems is needed to monitor the impact of large-scale cancer control programs. The development and funding of such a reporting network should be supported by the NCI Cancer Control Program. The required network can in part be built around the Comprehensive Cancer Research Centers that are being established.
d) To increase the efforts in cancer epidemiology, a selected number of population-based study centers will be developed and funded by the Demography Area (Biometry and Epidemiology Branches) NCI.

The table below summarizes the sources of support:

Type of Registry	Source of Support
Hospital - service oriented	Non-NCI
Comprehensive Cancer Research Center - treatment evaluation	NCI Grant
Community - monitoring of control programs	NCI Cancer Control Program
Epidemiology Research Center	NCI Demography Area

National Coordination. Before turning to a discussion of how the registry network should be coordinated to serve national program needs, it should be emphasized that the individual registries have their own goals and objectives. Activities at the national level should in no way diminish the initiative and enterprise of individual registry staffs in the development of their own study programs. In fact, the registry network may be viewed as an opportunity to extend the study facilities of individual registries; for some purposes the volume of experience at their disposal may not be sufficient, and arrangements for the local registry staff to tap the larger resources of the registry network to handle problems they have defined for investigation should be encouraged.

The National Cancer Institute, which must fund a substantial part of the cost of an expanded registry network, is the obvious candidate for the role of national coordinator, since the Biometry Branch has carried out a similar assignment in its collaboration with the End Results Group. The preparation of national descriptive data on incidence and end results and the management of the data resource pose no technical problems. This phase deals with well defined parameters and the data product in terms of tapes, tabulations and publications can be readily specified. Existing procedures for data collection and processing for the End Results Group and for the Third National Cancer Survey appear adequate and will require only minor modifications and adaptations. Measures to ensure quality control in all phases of work from abstracting of hospital charts to internal consistency checks of computer tapes require trivial extensions of established routines. The Biometry Branch has an organizational structure and staff that can discharge this responsibility. One section would be responsible for field liaison with participating registries and be concerned with all phases of work leading to the delivery of data tapes, including consultation on abstracting and coding problems and the maintenance of quality control procedures. The analyses of incidence and survival data tend to be specialized activities, and the Branch has two sections, one primarily concerned with the analysis of incidence data and applications to epidemiological studies and the other with analysis of patient survival and related prognostic factors.

The coordination of work to be carried out by population-based cancer study centers and comprehensive cancer research centers presents a completely new dimension for a national program. Each center will be engaged in a broad panorama of multidisciplinary research and training activities, which are not amenable to centralized direction and control. The existing model for data handling presented by the End Results Group is not relevant in this context. There is no reasonable alternative to delegating responsibility for planning and development to the several centers. However, some mechanism must be created to facilitate exchange of information among the research centers and to enable them to develop programs compatible with broad national goals. No organizational format to achieve these ends has been suggested or refined, but we suspect that the appropriate route is to establish a committee which will include the directors of the several research centers as members. The frequency of committee meetings and the type of meeting agenda are questions to which there are no preconceived answers. It would seem unwise to freeze a rigid committee program and structure at the outset, and an evolutionary approach which will identify useful committee activities as they emerge with time appears preferable.

An integrated network of registries and study centers that provides input on both incidence and patient survival should strengthen the use of tumor registries as a research tool. The existing compartmentalization of data collection activities in the United States ignores the fact that tumor induction and rate of tumor growth in the host are merely different facets of the carcinogenic phenomenon. Only by considering both types of information can we attack such problems as whether the forces which influence the rate of tumor induction in man persist past that point to affect the subsequent course of disease in the host. A paper presented at an international symposium on endresults of cancer therapy held in Norway in 1963 did attempt to review selected international comparisons of incidence and survival from this vantage point (5). The data on 7 sites assembled from 6 countries exhibited interesting site-specific patterns and suggested some models by which variable relationships between incidence and survival experience might arise. Proposals were advanced for further studies of breast and lung cancer along these lines, but to date they have remained unimplemented. One reason for the lack of action has been the inability of several countries, including the United States, to describe systematically the incidence-survival relationships for individual sites, and their variability within population groups covered by their registries. It is our hope that an augmented program of cancer registration and allied clinical and epidemiological studies in the United States will remedy this deficiency in part and provide a powerful impetus for studies that will make important contributions to knowledge on the etiology and treatment of cancer.

References

1. The Registrar-General's Statistical Review of England and Wales for the Two Years 1966-1967. Supplement on Cancer. London: H. M. S. O. 1972.
2. Preliminary Report, Third National Cancer Survey, 1969 Incidence. DHEW Publication No. (NIH) 72, 1971.
3. End Results in Cancer, Report No. 4. U. S. Dept. of Health, Education, and Welfare, Public Health Service. Washington, D. C.: U. S. Govt. Printing Office 1972.
4. HAENSZEL, W., LOURIE, W. I., Jr.: Quality control of data in a large-scale cancer register program. Krebs - Dokumentation und Statistik maligner Tumoren 25, 89 (1965).
5. HAENSZEL, W. M.: Contributions of End Results Data to Cancer Epidemiology. In: International Symposium on End Results of Cancer Therapy, Ed. Cutler, S. J., p. 21. National Cancer Institute Monograph 15. U. S. Dept. of Health, Education, and Welfare, Public Health Service. Washington, D. C.: U. S. Govt. Printing Office 1964.

The Evaluation of Data Collection Procedures—Assessment of Completeness

T.H.C. Barclay

Cancer registration is a procedure whereby selected information about all patients with cancer in a precisely defined population is brought together centrally. Its objectives, ideally, should be to gather reliable data which will permit the measurement of the cancer problem in the community and to determine trends in incidence rates; to provide indices for evaluating the progress made in bringing cancer under control, to evaluate the services provided to the patient with cancer, to ensure continued care of the patient and to promote epidemiological, laboratory and clinical research. The attainment of these objectives presupposes access to adequate demographic, clinical and other relevant reports from which the pertinent data can be drawn.

The degreee to which registries can attain all these objectives varies. It is almost certain, however, that none will succeed unless certain basic criteria are satisfied. The registry should operate within a precisely defined geographic area. The size and characteristics of its population should be known, preferably by census survey. Medical services should be readily available and widely used and the level of diagnostic validity should be high. The registry should have access to records concerning all individuals with cancer in every hospital and every admission to hospital, from all radiotherapy departments, clinics and private physicians' offices within the area. Copies of all pathology, cytology and autopsy reports with a cancer annotation should be made available. The registry should receive a copy of the notification of death of all residents who have been certified as dying with cancer.

The reporting to the registry by all these independent sources not only increases the probability that all patients with cancer will sooner or later be registered, but, in many instances, also results in more accurate and complete information than the registry would have received if records were submitted only once and by only one agency. Multiple reporting may be a cumbersome procedure, creating for the registry the problems of accurate sorting, checking and matching of the data from the various sources, but experience justifies it as an excellent means of case finding. In Norway, information is submitted from at least two sources for 80 percent of the patients reported to the registry.

There is no doubt that registries that are established in countries where notification of cancer is compulsary operate at a distinct advantage.

An alternative to registries as a means of gathering data concerning patients with cancer is the operation of population-based, comprehensive diagnostic and treatment cancer centres such as those operating in the provinces of Saskatchewan and Alberta in Canada. In Saskatchewan, for example, where cancer is a notifiable disease, all residents, who have, or are suspected to have, cancer are referred by their family physicians to the clinics of the Saskatchewan Cancer Commission for investigation, diagnosis and treatment. All these services, including the cost of drugs directed at the control of cancer, are paid for by the provincial government and not by the individual patient. In this way the financial barrier to early diagnosis and treatment is removed.

In Saskatchewan, legislation makes it mandatory for all tissues removed at every operative procedure, however minor, to be sent for histological examination and for all pathology reports with a cancer annotation to be submitted to the Commission. Copies of all death certificates relating to Saskatchewan residents are submitted for scrutiny and verification of all cancer diagnoses.

In their roles as case-finding organizations, the only difference between a well-organized registry and the type of comprehensive clinical cancer program described lies in the source of their data. The registries are dependent upon outside agencies for their information, while in cancer clinics, with the exception of death certificates, the data are internally generated. The clinical type of program has advantages over the cancer registry in that certain disciplines regarding clinical data collection can be imposed more readily upon its medical staff than would be tolerable to even the most cooperative physician or surgeon working independently in a hospital. An example of the detail with which clinical data can be gathered in a clinically oriented program is presented in Tables 1 - 6. The advantages of incorporating clinical data of this or similar type into the registry system are obvious.

Perhaps the risk of duplication of registration is lower in clinical programs than in registries, but regular editing checks are necessary even in a clinical program.

One criterion by which the quality of a cancer registry can be measured is the proportion of its registered patients who have been included on the evidence of death certificate diagnosis only. Another, which is also a measure of the quality of care given to patients with cancer in a community, is the proportion of diagnoses confirmed by histology.

With regard to registration based on death certificate diagnosis only, a survey of the report of almost twenty registries throughout the world suggests that a level of 5 percent is acceptable. The registry in Puerto Rico has a creditable record of reducing its registration from death certificates only from 25 percent in 1950 to 3 percent in 1965. Finland reports 4 percent and Norway and Saskatchewan 2 percent.

In 1950, only 43 percent of cancer diagnoses in Puerto Rico were confirmed histologically. Because of the influence of the cancer registry and an improvement of the medical services in general, by 1968 confirmation was obtained in 85 percent. Most registries report histological proof of diagnosis in 80 to 90 percent of their patients. This is an acceptable level if we bear in mind that most registries do not include cancer of the skin in their records.

The bulk of diagnoses are made on clinical, radiological or operative (without biopsy) judgements.

In the calculation of incidence rates, there is no difficulty in relating the number of patients who are recognized to have cancer to the whole population in its age and sex divisions. It may be pertinent at this stage, however, to enquire how different registries interpret the

Table 1

PROVINCE OF SASKATCHEWAN
CANCER COMMISSION

HISTORY

BREAST CANCER 077

SEQUENCE NUMBER	CLINIC NUMBER			
	DATE OF EXAMINATION	DAY	MONTH	YEAR
	DOCTOR NUMBER			

SYMPTOMS BREAST INVOLVED

D1 (FIRST R L) / D3 (SUBSEQ R L)

01	NONE
02	LUMP IN BREAST
03	EXTRA MAMMARY
04	BREAST PAIN
05	BREAST TENDERNESS
06	NIPPLE DISCHARGE (BLOOD)
07	NIPPLE DISCHARGE (NON-BLOOD)
08	RETRACTION OF NIPPLE
09	ECZEMA OF NIPPLE
10	ULCERATION OF NIPPLE
11	REDNESS OF SKIN
12	EDEMA OF BREAST
13	PUCKERING OF SKIN
14	ULCERATION OF SKIN
15	HARDNESS OF BREAST
16	PEAU D'ORANGE
17	INCREASE IN BREAST SIZE
18	DECREASE IN BREAST SIZE
19	DEFORMITY OF BREAST

D2 / D4

01	PLEURAL EFFUSION
02	ASCITES
03	LIVER ENLARGEMENT
04	BONE PAIN
05	PATHOLOGICAL FRACTURE
06	CEREBRAL SYMPTOMS
07	OTHER (SPECIFY)

SYMPTOMS AND SIGNS

D5 (MM YY)

01	DATE OF FIRST SYMPTOMS
02	DATE OF FIRST VISIT TO M.D.
03	DATE OF ADMISSION TO CLINIC

LUMP DISCOVERED

E1

01	NOT STATED
02	PATIENT UNAWARE OF LUMP
03	ACCIDENTALLY BY PATIENT
04	DURING SELF-EXAMINATION OF BREAST
05	BECAUSE OF PAIN
06	BECAUSE OF NIPPLE DISCHARGE
07	BY FAMILY PHYSICIAN
08	AT CANCER CLINIC
09	OTHER (SPECIFY)

BREAST TENDERNESS, PAIN

E2 — 1. TENDERNESS 2. PAIN 3. DURATION IN MONTHS (1: R L, 2: R L, 3)

01	NONE
02	BREAST INVOLVED
03	GENERALI
04	LOCALIZED
05	NO RELATION TO MENSTRUATION
06	USUALLY PREMEN. ONLY
07	DURATION PROLONGED
08	INCREASED SEVERITY

PREVIOUS BREAST PATHOLOGY

E3 (RIGHT BREAST: HISTOLOGY, YEAR) / E4 (LEFT BREAST: HISTOLOGY, YEAR)

01	NONE
02	ABSCESS
03	FIBROADENOMA
04	FIBROCYSTIC DISEASE
05	DUCT PAPILLOMA
06	ADENOSIS
07	EPITHELIOSIS
08	"OTHER LUMP" - DISAPPEARED
09	CANCER
10	NOT KNOWN

HISTOPATHOLOGY PRIOR TO TREATMENT AT CANCER CLINIC

SOURCE OF TISSUE

E5

01	DATE (DD MM YY)
02	NOT APPLICABLE
03	BREAST LUMP
04	SIMPLE MASTECTOMY
05	LYMPH NODE
06	SKIN NODULE
07	NIPPLE DISCHARGE
08	PLEURAL FLUID
09	PLEURAL BIOPSY
10	ASCITIC FLUID
11	SPUTUM
12	SALINE WASHING
13	BONE CORE
14	MARROW BIOPSY
15	LIVER BIOPSY

TISSUE OBTAINED BY

F1

01	CANCER CLINIC
02	ROSTER SURGEON
03	NON-ROSTER SURGEON
04	GENERAL PRACTITIONER

REPORT ON THIS TISSUE

F2

01	CANCER
02	PRECANCER
03	BENIGN
04	TISSUE UNSATISFACTORY
05	DOUBTFUL

MENSTRUAL HISTORY

F3

01	DATE OF LAST MENSTRUATION (DD MM YY)
	1. USUALLY 2. CHANGED TO 3. DURATION (MM)
02	MENSTRUATION - REGULAR
03	- IRREGULAR
04	FLOW (IN DAYS)
05	LOSS - SCANT
06	- MODERATE
07	- HEAVY
08	CYCLE (IN DAYS)
09	AGE AT MENARCHE
10	AGE AT MENOPAUSE
11	AGE AT HYSTERECTOMY
12	PRESENTLY PREGNANT
13	PRESENTLY LACTATING
14	POST-PARTUM NON-LACTATING (3 MONTHS)
15	NOT APPLICABLE

PREVIOUS HYSTERECTOMY

F4

01	NOT APPLICABLE
02	BOTH OVARIES REMOVED
03	ONE OVARY RETAINED
04	BOTH OVARIES RETAINED
05	UNCERTAIN
06	RADIATION CASTRATION
07	OTHER PELVIC RADIATION
08	DATE PERFORMED (DD MM YY)
09	HOSPITAL PERFORMED

OBSTETRICAL HISTORY

F5

01	NUMBER OF LIVE BIRTHS
02	NUMBER OF STILL BIRTHS
03	NUMBER OF MISCAR. AND ABORTIONS AND ECTOPIC
04	TOTAL PREGNANCIES
05	AGE AT FIRST PREGNANCY
06	AGE AT LAST PREGNANCY

MEDICATIONS

G1 — 1. PRESENT 2. PAST 3. DURATION IN MONTHS

01	NONE
02	ESTROGENS
03	ESTROGEN CREAMS
04	ORAL CONTRACEPTIVES
05	ANDROGENS
06	OTHER (SPECIFY)

BREAST FEEDING

G2 — 1. Nº OF CHILDREN 2. MONTH LACTATING

01	LESS THAN 2 WEEKS
02	LESS THAN 3 MONTHS
03	LESS THAN 6 MONTHS
04	6 MONTHS AND OVER
05	TOTAL

REASONS FOR NO BREAST FEEDING

LESS THAN 2 WEEKS

G3

01	LACKING MILK
02	ABNORMAL NIPPLES
03	BREAST INFLAMMATION
04	CHILD DID NOT THRIVE
05	CONCURRENT DISEASE
06	PHYSICIAN'S ADVICE
07	NO INFORMATION
08	BY CHOICE

MALE BREAST CANCER

G4

01	PREVIOUS GYNECOMASTA
02	PREVIOUS TESTICULAR PATHOL
03	PREVIOUS PROSTATIC PATHOL
04	PROLONGED ESTROGEN THERAPY
05	PREVIOUS CASTRATION
06	UNDESCENDED TESTIS

Table 1 (continued)

PROVINCE OF SASKATCHEWAN
CANCER COMMISSION

NOTES and OBSERVATIONS

99	SITE	SEQUENCE NUMBER	CLINIC NUMBER	EFFECTIVE DATE	DOCTOR NUMBER	SECTION
01						
02						
03						
04						
05						
06						
07						
08						
09						
10						
11						
12						
13						
14						
15						
16						
17						
18						
19						
20						
21						
22						

NOTE:

SHOULD YOU WISH TO HAVE THIS MEMO APPEAR

A. AT THE BEGINNING OF THE PATIENT PRINT OUT
WRITE ZEROS IN THE SITE AND SECTION.

B. AFTER A SPECIFIC SECTION
WRITE THE SITE AND SECTION AFTER
WHICH THE MEMO IS TO APPEAR.

Table 2

PROVINCE OF SASKATCHEWAN
CANCER COMMISSION

EXAMINATION

BREAST CANCER 077

SEQUENCE NUMBER	CLINIC NUMBER			
	DATE OF EXAMINATION	DAY	MONTH	YEAR
	DOCTOR NUMBER			

BREAST EXAMINATION

H1

Item	Code	R	L
BREAST SIZE - RIGHT = LEFT	01		
- RIGHT > LEFT	02		
- RIGHT < LEFT	03		
NO VISIBLE DEFORMITY	04		
PUCKERING OF SKIN	05		
PEAU D'ORANGE	06		
VISIBLE LUMP	07		
SKIN NODULE (BREAST ONLY)	08		
SKIN NODULE (BEYOND BREAST)	09		
SKIN REDNESS OVER BREAST	10		
SKIN ULCERATION OVER TUMOR	11		
OEDEMA OF BREAST	12		
BREAST DEFORMITY	13		

NIPPLES

H2

Item	Code	R	L	NONE
LEVEL NOT STATED	01			
LEVEL OF NIPPLES SAME	02			
RIGHT HIGHER THAN LEFT	03			
RIGHT LOWER THAN LEFT	04			
NORMALLY EVERTED	05			
NORMALLY INVERTED	06			
RETRACTION - NONE	07			
- PARTIAL	08			
- COMPLETE	09			
ECZEMA	10			
ULCERATION	11			
DISCHARGE - NONE	12			
- BLOOD	13			
- SEROUS	14			
- OTHER	15			
- SCANT	16			
- MODERATE	17			
- COPIOUS	18			

SKIN TETHERING OVER TUMOR

H3

Item	Code	R	L
NOT STATED	01		
NONE	02		
UP TO 25% OF TUMOR SURFACE	03		
25 TO 50% OF TUMOR SURFACE	04		
51 TO 75% OF TUMOR SURFACE	05		
OVER WHOLE TUMOR	06		

PEAU D'ORANGE

H4

Item	Code	R	L
NOT STATED	01		
NONE	02		
ONLY SKIN OVER LUMP	03		
BEYOND LUMP (WITHIN BREAST)	04		
OVER LUMP & BEYOND BREAST	05		
WHOLE BREAST	06		
WHOLE BREAST & BEYOND	07		

BREAST LUMP

J1

Item	Code	R	L
NO LUMP PALPABLE	01		
NUMBER OF BREAST LUMPS	02		
SITE OF LUMP - CENTRAL	03		
- WHOLE BREAST	04		
- CLOCK READING OF LUMP >	05		
- CLOCK READING OF LUMP <	06		
- DISTANCE FROM NIPPLE (cm) >	07		
- DISTANCE FROM NIPPLE (cm) <	08		
SIZE OF LUMP - LARGEST (cm) - MAX. AXIS	09		
- LARGEST (cm) - MIN. AXIS	10		
- SMALLEST (cm) - MAX. AXIS	11		
- SMALLEST (cm) - MIN. AXIS	12		
OUTLINE OF LUMP - NOT APPLICABLE	13		
- DISCRETE	14		
- POORLY DEFINED	15		

CONSISTENCY OF LUMP

J2

Item	Code	R	L
NOT STATED	01		
HARD	02		
FIRM	03		
SOFT	04		
FLUCTUANT	05		

FIXATION OF LUMP

J3

Item	Code	R	L
NOT STATED	01		
NO FIXATION	02		
TO SKIN	03		
TO NIPPLE	04		
TO PECTORAL FASCIA	05		
TO PECTORAL MUSCLE	06		
TO CHEST WALL	07		

TRANSILLUMINATION

J4

Item	Code	R	L
NOT DONE	01		
DARK SHADOW	02		
LIGHT SHADOW	03		
"HIGHLIGHT" OVER LUMP	04		
NO SHADOW	05		

BREAST TENDERNESS

J5

Item	Code	R	L
NONE	01		
ENTIRE BREAST	02		
OVER LUMP ONLY	03		
OVER BREAST - NOT OVER LUMP	04		

BREAST ULCERATION

H5

Item	Code	R	L
NONE	01		
NIPPLE	02		
WITHIN BREAST	03		
BEYOND BREAST	04		
DIMENSION OF ULCERATION (cms.) - MAX. AXIS	05		
- MIN. AXIS	06		

SKIN NODULES

K1

Item	Code	R	L
NONE	01		
IN CONTINUITY WITH TUMOR	02		
NOT IN CONTINUITY	03		
OVER BREAST ONLY	04		
BEYOND BREAST	05		
OPPOSITE CHEST WALL	06		
NECK	07		
BACK	08		
ABDOMINAL WALL	09		
SINGLE	10		
MULTIPLE	11		
OTHER REMOTE SITE	12		
SIZE LARGEST NODULE (cm) - MAX AXIS	13		
- MIN AXIS	14		

PALPABLE LYMPH NODES

K2

CODES ARE AS FOLLOWS:
1 -- NOT PALPABLE
2 -- PREVIOUSLY REMOVED
3 -- MOVEABLE
4 -- MATTED
5 -- FIXED TO CHEST WALL
6 -- TETHERED TO SKIN

Item	Code	1	2	3	4	5	6
RIGHT							
UPPER AXILLARY	01						
LOWER AXILLARY	02						
SUPRACLAVICULAR	03						
CERVICAL	04						
LEFT							
UPPER AXILLARY	05						
LOWER AXILLARY	06						
SUPRACLAVICULAR	07						
CERVICAL	08						

PALPABLE NODES CONSIDERED INVOLVED

K3

Item	Code	R	L	NONE
UPPER AXILLARY	01			
LOWER AXILLARY	02			
SUPRACLAVIC	03			
CERVICAL	04			
LYMPHOEDEMA ARM	05			

OTHER METASTASES CLINICAL ASSESSMENT

K4

Item	Code
OTHER BREAST	01
PLEURAL	02
PULMONARY	03
LIVER	04
ABDOMINAL (ASCITES)	05
OVARY	06
BONE	07
CEREBRAL	08

IMPRESSION BASED ON HISTORY AND CLINICAL EXAMINATION ONLY

K5

Item	Code	R	L
BENIGN	01		
PREMALIGNANT	02		
MALIGNANT	03		
UNCERTAIN	04		
N.A. POST OPERATIVE	05		

IF CONSIDERED MALIGNANT

Item	Code	R	L
STAGE 0	06		
STAGE 1	07		
STAGE 2	08		
STAGE 3	09		
STAGE 4	10		
NOT STAGED	11		

		T									N				M	
		SIT	0	1	2	3	4	5	6	7	0	1	2	3	0	1
R	12															
L	13															

Table 2 (continued)

PROVINCE OF SASKATCHEWAN
CANCER COMMISSION

NOTES and OBSERVATIONS

99	SITE	SEQUENCE NUMBER	CLINIC NUMBER	EFFECTIVE DATE	DOCTOR NUMBER	SECTION
01						
02						
03						
04						
05						
06						
07						
08						
09						
10						
11						
12						
13						
14						
15						
16						
17						
18						
19						
20						
21						
22						

NOTE:

SHOULD YOU WISH TO HAVE THIS MEMO APPEAR

A. AT THE BEGINNING OF THE PATIENT PRINT OUT
WRITE ZEROS IN THE SITE AND SECTION.

B. AFTER A SPECIFIC SECTION
WRITE THE SITE AND SECTION AFTER
WHICH THE MEMO IS TO APPEAR.

Table 3

PROVINCE OF SASKATCHEWAN CANCER COMMISSION

INVESTIGATIONS

BREAST CANCER 077

SEQUENCE NUMBER	CLINIC NUMBER	
	DATE OF EXAMINATION	DAY MONTH YEAR
	DOCTOR NUMBER	

LABORATORY INVESTIGATIONS AT TIME OF FIRST EXAMINATION

L1

Item	Code
NOT DONE	01
HAEMOGLOBIN (gr)	02
W B C	03
URINE ESTROGEN /24hours)	04
OTHERS (SPECIFY)	05

ESTROGEN STATUS BY VAGINAL SMEAR

L2

Item	Code
NOT APPLICABLE	01
NOT DONE	02
MAXIMAL EFFECT	03
MODERATE EFFECT	04
SLIGHT EFFECT	05
SLIGHT DEFICIENCY	06
MODERATE DEFICIENCY	07
MAXIMAL DEFICIENCY	08
IMPRESSION GAINED TO DATE re: HORMONAL STATUS	
ESTROGEN POSITIVE	09
ESTROGEN NEGATIVE	10

X-RAY INVESTIGATIONS AT TIME OF FIRST EXAMINATION

L3

Item	Code	R	L
BONES			
NOT DONE	01		
BONE METASTASES			
NONE	02		
SKULL	03		
SPINE	04		
STERNUM	05		
RIBS	06		
PELVIS	07		
UPPER LIMB	08		
LOWER LIMB	09		
SCAPULA	10		

TYPE BONE METASTASES

L4

Item	Code
OSTEOLYTIC	01
OSTEOBLASTIC	02
MIXED	03

CHEST

L5

Item	Code
NOT DONE	01
LUNGS NORMAL	02
PULMONARY METASTASES	03
PLEURAL METASTASES	04
PLEURAL EFFUSION	05
PULMONARY FIBROSIS	06
PLEURAL THICKENING	07
MEDIASTINAL ABNORMAL	08

MAMMOGRAPHY

L6

Item	Code	R	L
NOT DONE	01		
NORMAL	02		
CYST	03		
DUCT ECTASIA	04		
CYSTIC DISEASE	05		
FIBROADENOMA	06		
CANCER	07		
DOUBTFUL	08		
UNSATISFACTORY	09		
UNSUSPECTED LUMP FOUND	10		

AXILLARY NODES

M1

Item	Code	R	L
NOT VISUALIZED	01		
NOT INVOLVED	02		
CANCER	03		

SCAN

M2

1. LIVER - 2. BRAIN - 3. BREAST	Code	1	2	3
NOT DONE	01			
POSITIVE	02			
NEGATIVE	03			
EQUIVOCAL	04			

BONE SCAN

M3

Item	Code	R	L
NOT DONE	01		
NORMAL UPTAKE	02		
ABNORMAL UPTAKE			
SKULL	03		
SPINE	04		
STERNUM	05		
RIBS	06		
PELVIS	07		
UPPER LIMB	08		
LOWER LIMB	09		
SCAPULA	10		

IMPRESSION BASED ON HISTORY, CLINICAL EXAMINATION, LABORATORY AND X-RAY STUDIES

M4

Item	Code	R	L
BENIGN	01		
PREMALIGNANT	02		
MALIGNANT	03		
UNCERTAIN	04		
NOT APPLICABLE	05		

IF CONSIDERED MALIGNANT

Item	Code	R	L
STAGE 0	06		
STAGE 1	07		
STAGE 2	08		
STAGE 3	09		
STAGE 4	10		
NOT STAGED	11		

		T									N				M	
		SIT	0	1	2	3	4	5	6	7	0	1	2	3	0	1
R	12															
L	13															

Table 3 (continued)

PROVINCE OF SASKATCHEWAN
CANCER COMMISSION

NOTES and OBSERVATIONS

99	SITE	SEQUENCE NUMBER	CLINIC NUMBER	EFFECTIVE DATE	DOCTOR NUMBER	SECTION
01						
02						
03						
04						
05						
06						
07						
08						
09						
10						
11						
12						
13						
14						
15						
16						
17						
18						
19						
20						
21						
22						

NOTE:

SHOULD YOU WISH TO HAVE THIS MEMO APPEAR

A. AT THE BEGINNING OF THE PATIENT PRINT OUT
WRITE ZEROS IN THE SITE AND SECTION.

B. AFTER A SPECIFIC SECTION
WRITE THE SITE AND SECTION AFTER
WHICH THE MEMO IS TO APPEAR.

Table 4

PROVINCE OF SASKATCHEWAN CANCER COMMISSION

TREATMENT

BREAST CANCER 077

SEQUENCE NUMBER	CLINIC NUMBER			
	DATE OF EXAMINATION	DAY	MONTH	YEAR
	DOCTOR NUMBER			

FIRST PLANNED COURSE OF TREATMENT

REASON PRIMARY TREATMENT NOT GIVEN AT CANCER CLINIC — M5

AGE	01
CONCURRENT DISEASE	02
OTHER CANCER DIFFERENT SITE	03
CANCER TOO ADVANCED	04
PATIENT REFUSED TREATMENT	05
PATIENT'S DECISION TREATMENT ELSEWHERE	06
PATIENT REFERRED ELSEWHERE	07
PREVIOUS ADEQUATE TREATMENT ELSEWHERE	08
PREVIOUS INADEQUATE TREATMENT ELSEWHERE	09
PATIENT PARTIALLY TREATED ELSEWHERE	10
NOT APPLICABLE	11

PREVIOUS TREATMENT GIVEN ELSEWHERE

N1

IN SASKATCHEWAN	01
OUT OF PROVINCE	02
EXCISION BIOPSY LUMP	03
QUADRANT RESECTION	04
SIMPLE MASTECTOMY	05
MODIFIED RADICAL MASTECTOMY	06
RADICAL MASTECTOMY	07
OOPHORECTOMY (BILAT)	08
RADIATION CASTRATION	09
PREOPERATIVE RADIATION	10
POSTOPERATIVE RADIATION	11

INTENTION OF PLANNED TREATMENT

N2

NO TREATMENT	01
NOT STATED	02
"FOR CURE"	03
PALLIATION	04
PAIN RELIEF ONLY	05
GROWTH RESTRAINT	06

TREATMENT ADVISED

N3

SURGERY	01
PREOPERATIVE RADIATION	02
POSTOPERATIVE RADIATION	03
HORMONES	04
CHEMOTHERAPHY	05
OTHER (SPECIFY)	06

RADIATION THERAPY PREOPERATIVE

(REASONS FOR) — N4

NOT APPLICABLE	01
LARGE SIZE OF TUMOR	02
EXTENT SKIN INVOLVEMENT	03
SKIN INVOLVEMENT & ULCERATION	04
PROJECT	05
OTHER (SPECIFY)	06

RADIATION THERAPY PREOPERATIVE

TREATMENT GIVEN — N5

		R	L
PRIMARY SITE	01		
REGIONAL LYMPH NODES	02		
RADIATION CASTRATION	03		
WITH HYPERBARIC O_2	04		
RADIOTHERAPIST CODE NUMBER	05		

HORMONE THERAPY

(REASONS FOR) — N6

NOT APPLICABLE	01
LOCAL EXTENT OF DISEASE	02
REMOTE SPREAD OF DISEASE	03
ADVANCED AGE - NO SURGERY	04
CONCURRENT DISEASE - NO SURGERY	05

SURGERY

P1

		R	L
SURGEON CODE NUMBER	01		
DATE OF SURGICAL TREATMENT	02 (DD MM YY)		
BIOPSY	03		
EXCISION OF LUMP ONLY	04		
QUADRANT RESECTION	05		
SIMPLE MASTECTOMY	06		
HALSTED RADICAL MASTECTOMY	07		
MODIFIED RADICAL MASTECTOMY	08		
BILATERAL OOPHORECTOMY	09		
BILATERAL ADRENALECTOMY	10		
HYPOPHYSECTOMY	11		
OTHER (SPECIFY)	12		

HISTOLOGY

PRIMARY TUMOR — P2

		R	L
NONE	01		
ADENOCARCINOMA	02		
UNDIFFERENTIATED CANCER	03		
INFLAMMATORY CANCER	04		
MEDULLARY CANCER	05		
MUCOUS CANCER	06		
DUCT CANCER (INFILT)	07		
DUCT CANCER (NO INFILT)	08		
EPIDERMOID CANCER	09		
CYSTOSARCOMA PHYLLOIDES	10		
FIBROSARCOMA	11		
LIPOSARCOMA	12		
LYMPHOSARCOMA	13		
LOBULARSARCOMA	14		
MULTIPLE PRIMARY IN BREAST	15		
OTHER (SPECIFY)	16		

LYMPH NODE INVOLVEMENT

AXILLA — P3

		R	L
AX NODES NOT REMOVED	01		
NO INVOLVEMENT	02		
UPPER NODES INVOLVED	03		
LOWER NODES INVOLVED	04		
AXILLARY FAT INVOLVED	05		
SINUS HISTIOCYTOSIS	06		
PARASTERNAL			
NOT REMOVED	07		
CONTAIN TUMOR	08		
CONTAIN NO TUMOR	09		
SUPRACLAVICULAR			
NOT REMOVED	10		
CONTAIN TUMOR	11		
CONTAIN NO TUMOR	12		

BLACKS GRADING ATYPIA

P4

		R	L
A.P.	01		
A	02		
B	03		
C	04		
D	05		
SUM CALC.	06		

POSTOPERATIVE STAGING OF TUMOR

P5

		R	L
STAGE 0	01		
STAGE I	02		
STAGE 2	03		
STAGE 3	04		
STAGE 4	05		
NOT STAGED	06		

		T									N				M	
		SIT	0	1	2	3	4	5	6	7	0	1	2	3	0	1
R	07															
L	08															

Table 4 (continued)

PROVINCE OF SASKATCHEWAN
CANCER COMMISSION

NOTES and OBSERVATIONS

99	SITE	SEQUENCE NUMBER	CLINIC NUMBER	EFFECTIVE DATE	DOCTOR NUMBER	SECTION
01						
02						
03						
04						
05						
06						
07						
08						
09						
10						
11						
12						
13						
14						
15						
16						
17						
18						
19						
20						
21						
22						

NOTE:

SHOULD YOU WISH TO HAVE THIS MEMO APPEAR
A. AT THE BEGINNING OF THE PATIENT PRINT OUT
WRITE ZEROS IN THE SITE AND SECTION.
B. AFTER A SPECIFIC SECTION
WRITE THE SITE AND SECTION AFTER
WHICH THE MEMO IS TO APPEAR.

Table 5

PROVINCE OF SASKATCHEWAN CANCER COMMISSION

RADIOTHERAPY

BREAST CANCER 077

SEQUENCE NUMBER	CLINIC NUMBER			
	DATE OF EXAMINATION	DAY	MONTH	YEAR
	DOCTOR NUMBER			

RADIATION THERAPY INTENTION OF TREATMENT — P6

NO RADIATION THERAPY	01
FOR CURE	02
PALLIATION	03
PAIN RELIEF ONLY	04
GROWTH RESTRAINT	05
OTHER (SPECIFY)	06

HISTORY OF RADIATION THERAPY PRIOR TO SCC ADMISSION — Q1

LEFT

		DAY	MONTH	YEAR
DATE TREATMENT STARTED	01			
DATE TREATMENT FINISHED	02			
TOTAL DOSE (RADS)	03			

RIGHT

		DAY	MONTH	YEAR
DATE TREATMENT STARTED	04			
DATE TREATMENT FINISHED	05			
TOTAL DOSE (RADS)	06			

DETAILED PLAN OF TREATMENT FIELDS — Q2

		R	L
PARASTERNAL	01		
AXILLA	02		
SUPRACLAVICULAR	03		
TUMOUR ONLY	04		
WHOLE BREAST	05		
CHEST WALL (ENTIRE)	06		
CHEST WALL (MEDIUM)	07		
CHEST WALL (SMALL)	08		
QUADRATE TECHNIQUE	09		
SINGLE FIELD	10		
PARALLEL PAIR	11		
PARALLEL PAIR TANGENITIAL	12		
WEDGE FILTERS	13		
BEAM TRIMMERS	14		
CIRCULAR	15		
IRREGULAR	16		

FIELD SIZE (cms)	17	
DIAMETER IN CIRCULAR FIELD	18	(cms)
TOTAL AREA (IRREGULAR FIELD)	19	(sq. cm)
FOR CASTRATION	20	

EQUIPMENT AND SOURCE — Q3

K.V. 120	01
K.V. 220	02
K.V. 280	03
K.V. 400	04
Co 60	05
BETATRON	06
VOLTAGE K.V.	07
VOLTAGE M.E.V.	08
MILLIAMPS	09
H.V.L. Al.	10
H.V.L. Cu.	11
H.V.L. Pb.	12

C.M.S.

F.S.D.	13
S.S.D.	14
F.T.D.	15
S.T.D.	16

RADIATION THERAPY AT SCC — Q4

RADIOTHERAPIST CODE Nº	01

TOTAL DOSE (RADS)

TO TUMOR	02
TO SKIN	03
NUMBERS OF TREATMENTS	04

DURATION OF TREATMENT

		DAY	MONTH	YEAR
DATE TREATMENT BEGUN	05			
DATE TREATMENT ENDED	06			

RADS

MAXIMUM TUMORI DOSE	07
MINIMUM TUMOR DOSE	08
MAXIMUM SKIN DOSE	09
INTEGRAL DOSE	10

INTRACAVITARY OR INTERSTITIAL — Q5

SITE

		R	L
NONE	01		
CHEST WALL	02		

SOURCE

RADIUM	03
RADIOACTIVE GOLD GRAINS	04
RADON	05
COBALT	06
CESIUM	07
TANTALLUM	08
COLLOIDAL GOLD	09
CHROMIUM PHOSPH. P-32	10

TYPE OF APPLICATION — Q6

IMPLANT	01
MOULD	02
INTRACAVITARY	03
EXTRAPLEURAL PARASTERNAL	04
OTHER (SPECIFY)	05

TECHNIQUE — R1

LINE SOURCE	01
SINGLE PLANE	02
SANDWICH	03
VOLUME	04
FLUID (INTRACAVITARY)	05
OTHER (SPECIFY)	06

SIZE OF FIELD — R2

SQUARE CM	01
CUBIC CM	02

TUMOR DOSE GIVEN — R3

MAXIMUM (RADS)	01
MINIMUM (RADS)	02
INTEGRAL (RADS)	03

DURATION OF TREATMENT

HOURS	04
DAYS	05

NUMBER OF APPLICATIONS OR INSERTIONS

06
07

DATES OF TREATMENT

		DAY	MONTH	YEAR
STARTED	08			
ENDED	09			
PERMANENT INSERTION	10			

RADIOTHERAPY FOR: — R4

RESIDUAL DISEASE (LOCAL)	01

RADIOTHERAPY FOR METASTASES TO

NONE	02
SKIN	03
REGIONAL LYMPH NODES	04
DISTANT LYMPH NODES	05
BONE	06
LUNG	07
PLEURA	08
PERITONEUM	09
BRAIN	10
OTHER BREAST	11

RADIATION ABLATION OF — R5

NONE	01
OVARIES	02
PITUITARY	03

Table 5 (continued)

PROVINCE OF SASKATCHEWAN
CANCER COMMISSION

NOTES and OBSERVATIONS

99	SITE	SEQUENCE NUMBER	CLINIC NUMBER	EFFECTIVE DATE	DOCTOR NUMBER	SECTION
01						
02						
03						
04						
05						
06						
07						
08						
09						
10						
11						
12						
13						
14						
15						
16						
17						
18						
19						
20						
21						
22						

NOTE:

SHOULD YOU WISH TO HAVE THIS MEMO APPEAR
A. AT THE BEGINNING OF THE PATIENT PRINT OUT
WRITE ZEROS IN THE SITE AND SECTION.
B. AFTER A SPECIFIC SECTION
WRITE THE SITE AND SECTION AFTER
WHICH THE MEMO IS TO APPEAR.

Table 6

PROVINCE OF SASKATCHEWAN CANCER COMMISSION

TREATMENT RESULTS

BREAST CANCER 077

SEQUENCE NUMBER	CLINIC NUMBER	
	DATE OF EXAMINATION	DAY MONTH YEAR
	DOCTOR NUMBER	

RESULTS OF PLANNED TREATMENT

S2

PLANNED TREATMENT CURATIVE	01
MODIFIED TREATMENT PALLIATIVE	02
PLANNED TREATMENT PALLIATIVE	03
MODIFIED TREATMENT CURATIVE	04

REASON FOR MODIFICATION IN PLANNED RADIOTHERAPY

S3

NO MODIFICATION MADE	01
PATIENT DIED POSTOPERATIVELY	02
TREATMENT DELAY DUE TO DELAYED HEALING	03
TREATMENT DELAY DUE TO WOUND INFECTION	04
DELAY DUE TO FLUID UNDER FLAPS	05
GENERAL CONDITION OF PATIENT (CHANGE IN)	06
PATIENT REFUSED RADIATION	07
CLINICAL IMPRESSION OF STAGE INCORRECT	08
DISEASE MORE EXTENSIVE THAN ASSESSED	09
DISEASE LESS EXTENSIVE THAN ASSESSED	10
PATIENT REFUSED RADIATION CASTRATION	11
OTHER REASON FOR NO RADIATION CASTRATION	12
OTHER (SPECIFY)	13

COMPLICATIONS OF RADIOTHERAPY

(WITHIN 30 DAYS)

S4

NONE	01
DRY DESQUAMATION OF SKIN	02
MOIST DESQUAMATION OF SKIN	03
ESOPHAGITIS	04
RADIATION SICKNESS	05
OTHER (SPECIFY)	06

REASONS FOR MODIFICATIONS IN SURGICAL TREATMENT PLAN

S5

NO MODIFICATION MADE	01
PATIENT DECLINED ADVISED TREATMENT	02
OPINION DIFFERENCE BETWEEN SURGEON AND CLINIC	03
ON EXTENT OF DISEASE	04
ON GENERAL CONDITION OF PATIENT	05
ON PHILOSOPHIC APPROACH TO TREATMENT	06
DISEASE MORE EXTENSIVE THAN ASSESSED	07
DISEASE LESS EXTENSIVE THAN ASSESSED	08
CHANGE IN CONDITION PATIENT DURING OPERATION	09
OOPHORECTOMY REFUSED BY PATIENT	10
OOPHORECTOMY WITHDRAWN BY SURGEON	11
NO OOPHORECTOMY-PROLONGED CONVALESCENCE	12
OTHER (SPECIFY)	13

MODIFIED SURGICAL TREATMENT GIVEN

S6

LOCAL EXCISION	01
QUADRANT RESECTION	02
SIMPLE MASTECTOMY	03
MODIFIED RADICAL MASTECTOMY	04
RADICAL MASTECTOMY	05
UNPLANNED BILATERAL OOPHORECTOMY DONE	06
PLANNED BILATERAL OOPHORECTOMY NOT DONE	07
OTHER (SPECIFY)	08

COMPLICATIONS OF SURGERY

(WITHIN 30 DAYS POST OPERATIVE)

T1

NONE	01
DEATH	02
WOUND INFECTION	03
WOUND DEHISCENCE	04
SLOW HEALING OTHER CAUSE	05
FLUID UNDER FLAP	06
PULMONARY EMBULUS	07
OTHER (SPECIFY)	08

CONDITION OF PATIENT AT END OF TREATMENT

(CLINICAL ASSESSMENT)

T2

DEATH AS RESULT OF CANCER	01
POSTOPERATIVE DEATH	02
DEATH RADIATION COMPLICATION	03
ALIVE WITH DISEASE CONTROLLED	04
ALIVE WITH DISEASE NOT CONTROLLED	05
ALIVE CONTROL DOUBTFUL	06
DIED WITH CONCURRENT DISEASE	07

Table 6 (continued)

PROVINCE OF SASKATCHEWAN
CANCER COMMISSION

NOTES and OBSERVATIONS

99	SITE	SEQUENCE NUMBER	CLINIC NUMBER	EFFECTIVE DATE	DOCTOR NUMBER	SECTION
01						
02						
03						
04						
05						
06						
07						
08						
09						
10						
11						
12						
13						
14						
15						
16						
17						
18						
19						
20						
21						
22						

NOTE:

SHOULD YOU WISH TO HAVE THIS MEMO APPEAR

A. AT THE BEGINNING OF THE PATIENT PRINT OUT
WRITE ZEROS IN THE SITE AND SECTION.

B. AFTER A SPECIFIC SECTION
WRITE THE SITE AND SECTION AFTER
WHICH THE MEMO IS TO APPEAR.

data collected on patients who present with simultaneous multiple cancers in different anatomical sites. They must either count the number of cancers identified and relate the total to the population, thereby counting cancers and not patients with cancer, or, in the overall calculation of cancer incidence, relate the number of patients with cancer (however many separate cancers each may have) to the total population. Lack of standardization in this regard between registries could make the interpretation of apparent differences in overall cancer incidence rates difficult.

In the calculation of incidence by site it would appear permissible to include each individual cancer and relate the total number to the defined population. However, different practices become evident when the disciplines of each registry are examined. More questions arise out of these differences, such as whether a patient who presents with simultaneous bilateral breast and ovarian cancer should be considered as one patient with cancer in both halves of a paired organ or as two patients with cancer in the same site, and whether the patient with multiple transitional cell cancers of the urinary bladder or with two or three separate cancers involving different levels of the colon should be considered as one patient with cancer of the urinary bladder or colon, or as the same number of patients as there are cancers. It is the practice in Saskatchewan to count patients with cancer and use this number in the calculation of overall incidence, to count the number of cancers in different and nonpaired organs and apply this number only in the site incidence, and where more than one cancer appears in the same organ, or in the two halves of a paired organ, to count the patient as one patient with cancer in that specific site. Specific detailed data are recorded, however, to permit studies on incidence, e.g. of bilateral cancer of the breast or ovary or multiple cancers in other single organs. This may be a trivial point, but it is introduced for the purpose of ensuring standardization in our reporting.

The responsibilities of a cancer registry should extend beyond that of establishing incidence rates within its own community. Reference was made earlier to three other objectives of registries, namely to provide indices for evaluating the progress made in bringing cancer under control, to evaluate the services provided to the patient with cancer and to ensure the continued care of the patient. In order to fulfill these objectives, the stage of the disease, the treatment given, and the response to treatment in terms of control of the disease and survival should also be recorded.

It is not clear from most registry reports what is meant by "stage at the time of diagnosis." In California it appears that staging is based upon histological evidence, as otherwise the category "in situ" would not be specified in their data proforma. In other registries staging may be based on clinical findings and not on histological evidence, even when this becomes available. Those which have adopted the T. N. M. system are required by the dsiciplines of the method to make their assessment on clinical and radiological grounds only for most sites of disease. Experience has shown, however, that in a significant proportion of cases clinical assessment of stage is inconsistent with the findings after histological tissue examination. Standardization would be possible only if all registries were to adopt the same staging criteria.

Most registries record treatment given in the general terms of surgery, radiotherapy, chemotherapy or combinations of two or more of these methods. Some are convinced that the evaluation of treatment achievement classified by differences in surgical procedure, by dosage and duration of drug therapy does not belong to the function of a central cancer registry. In the absence of more specific description, however, it would help in the assessment of the end results of definitive treatment if all registries included in their data bank a declaration of the intention of treatment, i.e. whether "for cure" or palliation.

In addition to their case finding activities, some registries have developed patient follow-up programs which permit the annual identification of patients who have previously been treated for cancer and are still alive but have clinical or other evidence of continuing recurrent or metastatic disease. Their assumption of the responsibility for the repeated clinical examination of patients bring these registries into line with the functions of cancer clinics and indicates their recognition that continued observation of patients is necessary for the effective control of the disease and the extension of useful life. The frequency with which the registries arrange for these review examinations varies, but few, it seems, conform to the routine of most cancer clinics. In cancer clinics all patients who have received treatment (and most who have not) attend for clinical examination at three-monthly intervals for three years, twice annually for the next two years and annually thereafter for as long as they live and remain well. With any evidence of recurrence or metastatic disease the follow-up examinations become more frequent. Although this may appear to be a rigid program, few patients object to the inconveniences of travelling what may be long distances and of the frequent examinations.Their willingness to participate in this review service is borne out in Saskatchewan by the fact that the loss to follow-up of more than 60,000 consecutive patients over a period of many years is less than 0.5 percent.

These follow-up programs have three useful by-products. The first, and not least, is the interest which they engender in the physicians and surgeons who have originally treated the patients in the continuous care of their patients, and the stimulus to their cooperation in the successful operation of the registry.

The second by-product is the ease with which prevalence rates for cancer can be calculated. There have been many attempts at accurate measurement of prevalence, but in the absence of follow-up clinics they have failed. The prevalence rate can be calculated by adding to the number of new patients discovered to have cancer each year those in whom the diagnosis has been established in previous years but who still survive with evidence of continuing, recurrent, or metastatic disease, and relating the total of these to the population of the community. In Saskatchewan the prevalence of cancer (including skin cancer) rose in the population at risk from 764 per 100,000 in 1946-1950 to 1495 per 100,000 in 1966-1970. The rate rose more sharply in males, from 809 in the first quinquennium to 1995 in the last. The corresponding rates for females were 709 and 1003.

The knowledge of both incidence and prevalence rates of cancer may be an indicator to the health authorities in the community of the facilities and resources needed to meet the needs of the patients with cancer.

The third advantage arising form the follow-up program is the greater accuracy and speed with which survival rates can be established. Uncertainty about the date and cause of death is reduced and the verification of death certificate diagnoses is facilitated.

Opinions vary as to the date from which survival of the patient should be calculated. Discussions with a number of directors of cancer programs in Canada revealed that survival was calculated in some organizations from the date of diagnosis, and in others from the date of the first day of treatment. If similar differences exist in the reporting systems of registries, perhaps it is time that some agreement is reached so that valid comparisons can be made. The End Results Section of the National Cancer Institute of the United States use the date of diagnosis as their starting point in the calculation of their observed and relative survival rates. This would presumably be universally acceptable if the dates of diagnosis and institution of treatment were synchronous, but often they are not. Adoption of the same criteria by our own registries has been suggested.

The last of the declared objectives of cancer registries is the promotion of research. Registries have made a significant contribution to epidemiology by indicating the geographic variations in the incidence of certain cancers. Perhaps we should now consider expanding our data banks to include surveys of the varying social, economic, nutritional and occupational conditions and environmental hazards relating to our population and in-depth studies on the influences of migration.

Our data may, in time, be designed to give pointers to the clinical identification of intrinsic conditions such as genetic predisposition, immunological impairment, hormonal effects and metabolic differences.

It may be that we are too modest in our evaluation of the potential of our registries to accumulate detailed data that will allow a better understanding of the disease we are all concerned with.

Administrative use of the Cancer Registry in the German Democratic Republic

H. Berndt

The functions and objectives of the cancer registry in the G. D. R. can only be properly understood in the light of some knowledge of the organization of cancer control in general. The cancer registry is a weapon in the fight against cancer and can be rightly understood only in this context. This survey is therefore divided into the following sections:

1. organization of cancer control;
2. methods of the cancer registry;
3. use in medical and social care of cancer patients;
4. use in regional and national planning and management

1. Organization of Cancer Control

The organization of cancer control laid down by law in 1952 has since been supplemented by additional regulations to the effect that the responsibility for cancer control lies with the councils of the approximately 200 counties and 15 regions. These bodies are under the jurisdiction of the Ministry of Health. An important step in cancer control was the Program for combatting cancer, issued in 1967, which gave scientifically founded recommendations to the region and county councils. For instance, the program provided for the establishment of cytodiagnostic laboratories in all counties, and emphasized the principle of a team approach to cancer by specialists from different fields. The current five-year plan includes gradual expansion of the prophylactic examination service.

The work of local and territorial medical officers is supported by a region and a county oncological commissioner. The county oncologist gives advice to the county physician in all questions of cancer control; as a rule, this is a part-time job only, and he is appointed by the county physician. He heads the county office for cancer control, which is responsible for the organization of prophylactic examinations, for the coordination of all activities, and for follow-up medical and social care of cancer patients. However, special diagnoses and therapy are carried out in specialized units of the hospitals.

The cancer registry is an important tool both in cancer control and in the supply of information to the region and county oncologists.

2. Methods of Cancer Registration

Every suspicion of or detection of a notifiable tumor and every death known or suspected to have resulted from such a tumor is subject to registration by the attending physician. The responsibility for registration rests on both external and resident physicians, doctors in hospitals and in private practice, clinicists and pathologists.

The list of notifiable tumors was extended in 1956, and now comprises both malignant (No. 140 - 208 I. C. D.) and benign intracranial tumors and the so-called precanceroses, of which carcinoma _in situ_ of the _cervix uteri_ (No. 234.0) is dominant in number and significance.

Tumor reports cover the following details:

- name, date of birth, and address of the affected or deceased patient;
- occupation and possible occupational carcinogenic influences;
- type and location of the tumor;
- stage of the tumor and degree of diagnostic certainty;
- date and nature of first tumor symptoms, date of first consultation, correct diagnosis and onset of treatment;
- method of treatment and results.

Every physician suspecting or diagnosing cancer fills in a simple registration form I. As a rule in-patient treatment is required, or at least referral to a specialist or a specialized institution, e.g. a radiological clinic. On completion of the first treatment the detailed registration form II is filled in by the specialist-staff; this form is almost as informative as a concise case history.

If additional treatment is required or recurrences or metastases occur, this must be noted on registration form III. At annual intervals the history of the patient is recorded on registration form IV. These checks are continued over a period of five years after successful treatment, i.e. if the patient is free of recurrences and/or metastases during this period. The follow-up period is extended for another five years from the date of any recurrence.

When a cancer patient dies or a notifiable tumor disease not been detected during the patient's lifetime is found at post mortem, the pathologist is required to report this and also to make a note on the death certificate. Thus, the death certificate gives information on tumors detected by the pathologist at post mortem.

All these reports are produced in duplicate and both copies are sent to the county cancer control office responsible for the residential area of the patient. One copy is retained in this office for use in further medical, social, and statistical work, while the other is sent to the central cancer registry in the central oncological institute.

3. Use in Medical and Social Care of Cancer Patients

The regulation requiring that a cancer report be given directly to the local office for cancer control is essential to the county oncologist's assumption of his full responsibility for improving cancer control.

Registration form I informs the county oncologist of any suspicion of cancer, giving him the chance to investigate each patient in whom cancer is suspected. Of course, this is basically the job of the attending physician, but sometimes a patient refuses a special examination that is recommended or a proposed treatment. A delay can also occur due to other factors that impede rapid clarification of the case. Sometimes a mother has difficulty in finding somebody to look after her children; in such cases, the county oncologist and the office's social worker may intervene and arrange for help. The county oncologist's task is to see that the cancer patient is examined and treated rapidly and competently.

When the treatment is finished, the county oncologist is informed by means of registration form II about the disease, its treatment, and the result; it is at this point that his responsibility for follow-up medical and social attendance begins.

Subsequent to his stay in hospital, the patient is granted a benefit payment for 6 months, which is renewed in the case of repeated treatment or during a long-lasting out-patient treatment. Patients with severe physical handicaps are entitled to nursing benefit, allowing them to pay for any additional help necessary. In cases of economic hardship further aid can be provided, e.g. fuel is sometimes supplied.

For follow-up attendance the county oncologist relies on cooperation with specialized medical services (tuberculosis, diabetes etc.), cooperation with practitioners in the given residential area, local nurses, and social organizations such as the Volkssolidarität and the Democratic Federation of Women. In this context, increasing importance has to be attributed to a state-run program providing additional care for elderly people, for most cancer patients - in the G. D. R. some 60% - are old age pensioners.

The county oncologist is also an arbitrator; he decides which patients will be sent for special health cures (about 10,000 patients go each year). He works together with a rehabilitation commission to facilitate re-integration into society and if possible into industry for as many cancer patients as possible.

The annual follow-up reports allow him to assess the success of treatment and to help where necessary.

All death certificates are sent to the county office for cancer control, which is thus also notified of such diseases that have not been recognized clinically; this enables the oncologist to make systematic efforts to improve diagnosis in his district.

In our opinion, decentralized registration of cancer patients is a very useful approach, and is essential if immediate care of the patients is to be provided.

4. Use in Regional and National Planning and Management

As already mentioned, one copy of each registration form is sent by the county office to the regional oncologist, who collects the copies and passes them to the central cancer registry. It is left to his discretion to make a separate interim analysis for his region; this, of course, is desirable because the central registry cannot fulfill all the requirements concerning statistical evaluation for each region.

For this reason, the handling of data varies in different regions according to interests and opportunities. I should like to illustrate the effectiveness of the cancer registry in the planning and implementation of measures for cancer control by reference to our studies in Berlin.

Analysis of the Prevalence of Cancer

The prevalence of cancer patients i.e. the number of persons being attended or monitored by the 8 district offices of the capital is counted at the end of the year (irrespective of whether they are clinically ill at the moment of counting or not), and thus important clinical data are obtained about fluctuation. We have made a first analysis up to the end of 1972, determining the age of patients and localization and stage of tumors. Some of the results were surprising: about one quarter of the cancer patients had basaliomas of the skin. We have since decided to replace individual registration of basaliomas and the long-term follow-up of these patients by a single count of newly detected cases. The administrative expenditure would otherwise be out of any proportion to its return, as these patients need extensive medical and social care only in exceptional cases.

In one district of Berlin with a population of about 100,000, we detected 654 cases of cancer (other than basaliomas and precanceroses). Of these, 470 were women, including 103 with breast cancer, 92 with cervical cancer, and 68 with other genital carcinomas. By contrast, only 35 bronchial carcinomas were counted in men. This analysis gives quite a different picture than data on cancer incidence. Most of the tumors were the relatively benign carcinomas of the female genitalia and the breast; carcinomas of lung and bronchi, which rapidly lead to death accounted for a far smaller proportion. Obviously, death occurs in the year of onset in many cases, which are consequently not represented in point prevalence.

To our knowledge, hardly any comparable data are available on cancer prevalence, yet such data would provide necessary information on where to start measures for rehabilitation.

Changes in Incidence

The central oncological institute publishes the number of new cases and some further details from the cancer registry in the yearbook "Das Gesundheitswesen der DDR." In the past, however, these publications have failed to give age-standardized figures, which makes direct comparison difficult.

We have therefore made a comparative investigation of cancer incidence in the G. D. R. for 1956 and 1966, the result of which has been published elsewhere (3). We present here some figures illustrating the changes for some frequent sites of cancer.

The incidence of carcinoma of the cervix remained almost constant (Fig. 1). In fact, the incidence may have declined, because of the overall tumor morbidity has increased slightly; this increase is due in part to improved methods of registration and detection rather than a real increase in cancer risk. If the incidence has remained constant for any single localization this probably means a reduced cancer risk.

Similar data were obtained for cancer of the stomach (Fig. 2). By contrast, morbidity rates for lung cancer have risen considerably. The risk for women is much lower than that for men, but nonetheless it rose by 100 percent for some age groups (Fig. 3).

In Berlin we have made a thorough study of cancer incidence in the two five-year periods 1960-1964 and 1965-1969, which has revealed an increase in all cancer diseases for both sexes. We have reason to doubt whether these data are a true reflection of the situation. In the first period (1960-1964) there was a great shortage of physicians, and the quality of medical care was certainly lower than it is today. It seems probable that in many cases physicians failed to report a tumor even when the disease had been established or was thought to exist (Table 1 and 2).

Fig.1

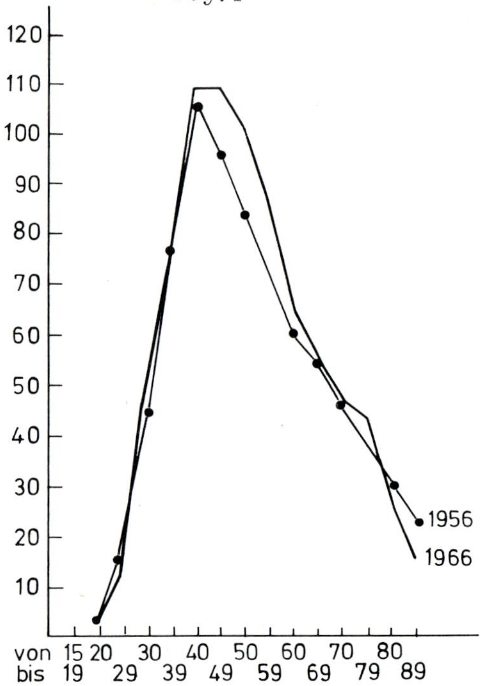

Fig.2

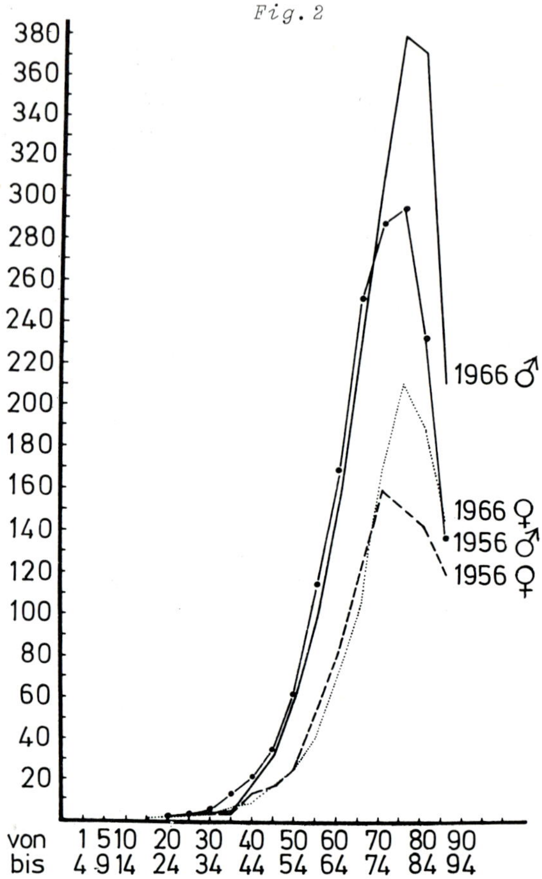

Fig. 1. Incidence per 100,000 / year of cancer of the cervix uteri (I.C.D. No. 180) in the G.D.R., 1956 and 1966, female by age

Fig. 2. Incidence per 100,000 / year of stomach cancer (I.C.D. No. 151) in the G.D.R., 1956 and 1966, by age and sex

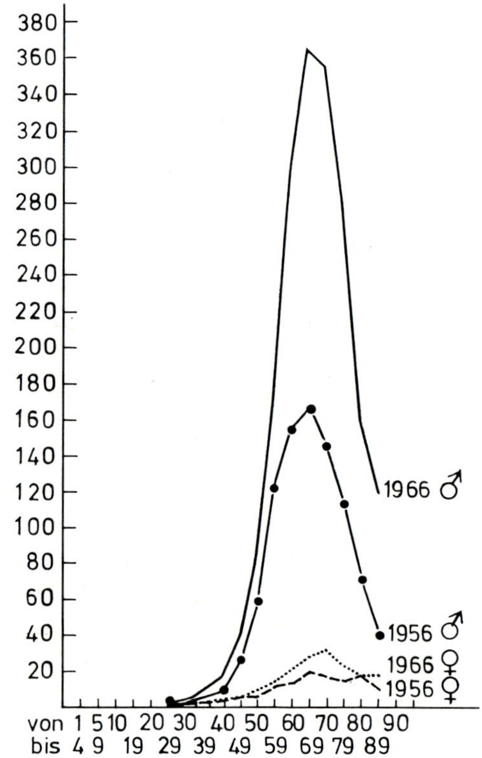

Fig. 3. Incidence per 100,000 / year of lung cancer (I.C.D. No. 162,1) in the G.D.R., 1956 and 1966, by age and sex

Some tumor localizations were found to deviate from this general trend, i.e. their incidence remained constant in comparison to the slight increase or increased more steeply than the general trend. For instance, the incidence of cancer of the cervix uteri and of the stomach has declined, while that of other cancers (e.g. carcinoma of the colon) has increased.

Regional Differences in Cancer Frequency

For malignant tumors with high fatality, mortality figures can be used instead of morbidity figures in the assessment of cancer risk and the analysis of regional differences. In an earlier study we established considerable regional differences in the incidence of gastrointestinal cancer in the G. D. R. (2) (Fig. 4).

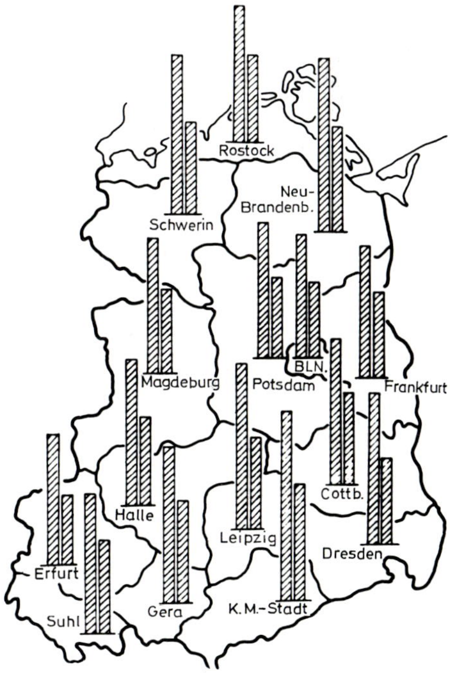

Fig. 4. Age-adjusted annual incidence of stomach cancer (I.C.D. No.151) per 100,000 in the regions of the G.D.R. in 1958-1960 (from BERNDT and WILDNER)

We have extended this study to the investigation of mortality rates for gastric cancer, cancer of the colon and rectum, and also cancer of the cervix uteri and the mammary gland. Figures for the 10-year period 1960-69 were not available for each year and county, but were usually contained for at least 7 or 8 years for each of the localizations mentioned. Because the regional population structure is different, and varied considerably over the period investigated, particularly as a result of migration to industrial centers, it was necessary to establish an age standardization. In order to give a lucid presentation of the results, the mortality for the G. D. R. was set to 100, which facilitates rapid comparison between the regions (Table 3).

Table 1 a. Incidence of malignant neoplasms per 100,000 of same age, male, 1960-1964, Berlin, capital of G.D.R.

	I.C.D.	Age groups (5-years classes)																	
	No.	0-	5-	10-	15-	20-	25-	30-	35-	40-	45-	50-	55-	60-	65-	70-	75-	80-	All
Lip	140								1.0	3.4	1.0	3.7	2.1	4.4	8.7	4.4	6.5	11.3	2.0
Tongue	141								1.0			2.4	1.0	5.6	1.7	1.1	14.6	6.8	1.3
Salivary glands	142					1.0	1.0				1.0	1.8	2.6	1.9	4.3	1.1		4.5	1.0
Mouth	143-145										1.0	0.6	1.0	2.5	3.5	7.6	1.6	2.3	0.9
Pharynx	146-149		0.7			0.5	0.5		2.0	1.1	2.9	4.3	4.7	7.5	9.6	12.1	17.9	6.8	3.2
Mesophagus	150									1.1	2.9	4.9	7.3	7.5	19.1	33.0	37.3	36.3	5.6
Stomach	151						1.5	2.6	2.9	9.1	18.6	50.0	63.0	111.9	154.5	208.9	231.7	167.9	43.7
Small intestine	152								1.0		2.0	1.2		1.2	2.6	1.1	4.9		0.6
Colon	153	0.5			0.7	0.5		1.3	2.9	6.8	7.8	11.0	19.3	30.0	40.8	53.9	60.0	74.9	12.7
Rectum	154				0.7		1.0	1.3	2.9	1.1	3.9	11.6	17.2	34.4	46.0	64.9	51.9	61.3	12.7
Liver	155	0.5		0.8						1.1	2.0	3.1	6.2	9.4	13.9	14.3	21.1	13.6	3.7
Gall bladder	156									1.1	1.0	4.3	2.6	10.6	16.5	29.7	19.4	27.2	4.4
Pancreas	157							1.3	1.0	1.1	4.9	6.1	10.9	15.6	21.7	15.4	25.9	18.2	5.6
Other digestive organs	158-159						0.5		1.0			1.8	1.0		1.7	3.3	3.2		0.6
Nose, Sinuses	160				0.7							1.8	1.6	1.9	0.9	3.3	8.1	9.1	1.0
Larynx	161							0.7	1.0	1.1	7.8	6.7	23.4	34.4	39.1	26.4	14.6	9.1	8.9
Trachea, Bronchus	162						1.0	4.6	3.8	12.5	52.0	86.6	181.1	277.5	360.1	287.0	186.3	103.5	80.6
Pleura	163.0											0.6	3.1	0.6	4.3	4.4	1.6		0.8
Mediastinum	163.1											0.6	3.1	1.9	1.7	2.2	1.6		0.7
Bone	170	1.1	0.7		1.4	0.5	1.0	0.7	1.0		1.0	3.1	3.6	2.5	5.2	7.7	11.3		2.0
Connective tissue	171	0.5			0.7			0.7		1.1	1.0	1.8	2.1	3.1	3.5	1.1	3.2		1.0
Melanoma, Skin	172, 173		1.3		2.9	5.1	5.6	8.5	12.5	19.4	58.0	45.1	68.2	86.9	116.3	148.4	205.8	263.2	42.9
Breast	174										2.0			1.9	1.7	6.6	6.5	2.3	0.8
Prostata	185										1.0	6.1	16.7	55.6	99.8	184.7	202.5	208.8	27.5
Testis	186	0.5			0.7	4.6	7.6	3.3	6.7	6.8	3.9	1.8	2.1	1.3	0.9	4.4		2.3	2.8
Other male sex organs	187							0.7		2.3		1.8	4.2	3.1	3.5	3.3	3.2	6.8	1.3
Urinary bladder	188		0.7						1.0	1.1	5.9	9.8	20.3	30.0	50.3	51.7	37.3	45.4	11.3
Kidney	189	2.1				0.5	0.5		1.0		6.9	7.3	14.1	15.0	19.1	14.3	17.8	18.2	5.7
Eye	190	1.1			0.7		0.5	0.7			2.9	4.3	2.6	3.7	2.6	1.1	3.2	2.3	1.4
Brain	191	3.2	3.9		1.4	3.2	2.6	3.3	4.8	2.3	7.8	9.2	10.0	8.1	4.3	2.2	8.1		4.6
Nervous system	192				0.7		0.5		1.0		1.0				1.7				0.2
Thyroid	193					0.5		0.7	1.9	1.1		1.2	1.0	2.5	0.9	1.1	3.2		0.7
Other endocr. glands	194	0.5						0.7				1.2	1.0		0.9	1.1		4.5	0.4
Other localization	195-199	0.5					0.5	0.7	2.9		2.9	3.7	8.3	11.9	9.5	16.5	9.7	4.5	3.7
Lympho-a. ret. sarcoma	200			0.8	2.2	1.4	2.6	2.6	1.0		2.0	1.8	5.2	3.1	6.9	8.8	11.3	6.8	2.7
Lymphogranulomatosis	201		0.6	2.3		3.7	3.6	2.6	1.0	2.3	1.0	3.7	4.7	3.7	6.1	2.2	3.2	2.3	2.6
Other lymph. tumors	202					1.4		0.6	1.9	1.1		1.8	1.0	1.9	5.2	3.3	3.2		1.1
Multiple myeloma	203								1.0		2.0	4.9	3.1	4.4	3.5	7.7	4.9	2.3	1.7
Acute lymph. leukemia	204.0	1.1				1.4						0.6	1.0	1.9	3.5	1.1	4.9	2.3	0.9
Chron. lymph. leukemia	204.1	0.5									2.9	3.1	7.3	10.6	13.0	12.1	13.0	15.9	3.5
Acute myel. leukemia	205.0	1.6			0.7		0.5	1.3			2.0		1.6	1.9		1.1	4.9		0.8
Chron. myel. leukemia	205.1		0.7	1.5	1.4	0.5	1.5	0.7	2.9	2.3	2.0	1.8	2.1	3.1	4.3	2.2	3.2		1.7
Other acute leukemia	207.0	0.5																	0.04
Other chron. leukemia	207.1	0.5																	0.04

Table 1 b. Incidence of malignant neoplasms per 100,000 of same age, male, 1965-1969, Berlin, capital of G.D.R.

	I.C.D. No.	Age groups (5-year classes) 0-	5-	10-	15-	20-	25-	30-	35-	40-	45-	50-	55-	60-	65-	70-	75-	80-	All
Lip	140							0.5	0.6	0.9	1.2	4.1	3.3	2.9	5.6	8.9	5.6	7.1	1.6
Tongue	141									0.9		1.0	3.9	5.3	4.0	8.9	5.6	11.8	1.6
Salivary glands	142	0.5				1.2	0.8	1.5	0.6	1.9	1.2		3.3	7.7	3.2	5.1	7.5		1.8
Mouth	143-145						0.4				1.2	3.1	3.9	4.1	7.2	6.4	7.1		1.4
Pharynx	146-149							0.9	0.6	2.8	3.5	6.1	8.5	12.4	11.2	10.2	15.1	7.1	3.4
Mesophagus	150									1.9	5.8	6.1	12.5	15.3	25.6	17.9	24.4	61.2	6.0
Stomach	151				0.7		0.8	1.9	2.5	13.2	21.9	51.0	83.5	128.4	179.4	228.4	317.0	369.7	48.9
Small intestine	152				0.7			0.5				1.0	0.7	1.8	5.6	1.3		4.7	0.7
Colon	153			0.6	0.7		1.3	1.5	3.8	10.4	12.7	15.3	25.0	47.1	69.7	81.7	114.4	113.0	18.0
Rectum	154						0.8	1.0		3.8	4.6	18.4	27.6	39.5	72.9	97.0	106.9	122.5	17.4
Liver	155							0.5		3.8	5.8	8.2	13.8	24.7	40.0	38.3	48.8	33.0	8.4
Gall bladder	156							0.5		0.9	2.3	5.1	9.9	17.1	27.2	38.3	80.7	49.5	7.6
Pancreas	157								1.3	3.8	8.1	14.3	21.7	33.0	36.8	45.9	41.3	49.5	10.1
Other digestive organs	158-159	1.4				0.6			0.6			3.1	0.7	2.9	3.2	1.3	3.8		0.9
Nose, Sinuses	160	0.5										1.0	1.3	5.9	4.8	1.3	1.9		0.9
Larynx	161						0.4	1.0	1.9	2.8	5.8	15.3	21.0	31.2	39.2	33.2	24.4	23.6	8.9
Trachea, Bronchus	162					0.6	0.8	2.4	7.5	16.0	56.5	113.2	226.8	417.1	546.1	614.9	506.5	346.2	118.6
Pleura	163.0							0.5			2.3	1.0	1.3	4.1	3.2	6.4	9.4	4.7	1.2
Mediastinum	163.1								0.6		1.2		1.3	4.1	3.2	3.8	5.6	2.4	0.9
Bone	170		0.5		2.9	1.2	1.3	1.0	1.3	1.9		4.1	3.9	4.1	8.8	7.7	11.3	14.1	2.6
Connective tissue	171					1.2	0.4	1.5	0.6		2.3	2.0	5.9	1.2	1.6	3.8	5.6	2.4	1.3
Melanoma, Skin	172,173					3.7	4.6	11.2	15.0	31.1	30.0	75.5	89.4	114.3	131.3	222.0	230.7	310.8	46.9
Breast	174							1.0			1.2	1.0		1.8	4.0	12.8	3.8	2.4	1.0
Prostata	185						0.4				2.3	9.2	23.0	66.6	118.5	214.3	324.5	388.5	34.1
Testis	186	0.9			4.4	5.6	12.6	9.7	4.4	3.8	3.5	1.0	1.3	2.4		6.4	1.9		3.9
Other male sex organs	187							0.5	0.6	0.9		3.1	2.0	3.5	4.8	6.4	11.3	9.4	1.5
Urinary bladder	188				0.7	0.6		0.5	2.5	3.8	10.4	15.3	23.7	56.6	77.7	88.0	84.4	77.7	17.2
Kidney	189	0.5						0.5	1.3	6.6	9.2	18.4	17.1	24.2	39.2	39.6	41.3	54.2	9.6
Eye	190	1.4	0.5				0.8	1.5	1.3		1.2		1.3	2.9	4.8	1.3	3.8		1.2
Brain	191	2.3	4.1	1.3	3.7	6.2	2.9	8.8	8.1	2.8	13.8	11.2	15.8	18.9	24.0	10.2	11.3	30.6	8.7
Nervous system	192	0.5	0.5	0.6	0.7	1.2	0.4		1.9			2.0	1.3	1.2	0.8		1.9		0.8
Thyroid	193						0.8		1.3	1.9	1.2	1.0	0.7	1.2	3.2	5.1		2.4	0.8
Other endocr. glands	194	1.4					0.4	1.0	0.6	2.8	1.2	1.0	2.0	1.8	1.6	3.8	3.8		1.0
Other localization	195-199				0.7		0.4		1.3	4.7	4.6	2.0	9.9	14.1	22.4	21.7	20.6	25.9	5.0
Lympho-a. ret. sarcoma	200	0.5	1.0	1.3	2.2	0.6	0.8	1.5	2.5	2.8	2.3	4.1	9.2	8.2	8.0	5.1	13.1	7.1	3.3
Lymphogranulomatosis	201		2.0	0.6	0.7	5.6	5.9	3.9	3.8	2.8	1.2	8.2	5.3	2.4	8.8	1.3	3.8	7.1	3.6
Other lymph. tumors	202	0.9						0.5	1.3	0.9	1.2		2.0	0.6		2.6	5.6	4.7	1.8
Multiple myeloma	203								0.6			1.0	3.3	7.7	6.4	16.6	15.0	2.4	2.1
Acute lymph. leukemia	204.0	4.1	1.5	0.6	1.5		0.8	1.5	0.6	1.9		5.1	5.3	2.9	8.0	8.9	9.4	11.8	2.8
Chron. lymph. leukemia	204.1			0.6				0.5	0.6		3.5	3.1	6.6	7.7	10.4	14.0	24.4	28.3	3.4
Acute myel. leukemia	205.0	2.3	0.5	1.3	0.7	1.2		1.0	0.6		1.2	2.0	2.0	1.2	2.4	5.1	13.1	7.1	1.6
Chron. myel. leukemia	205.1	0.5				3.7	0.8			0.9		2.0	3.3	3.5	4.0	8.9	9.4	2.4	1.7
Other acute leukemia	207.0	0.9	0.5															2.4	0.2
Other chron. leukemia	207.1	0.5											0.7						0.1

Table 2 a. Incidence of malignant neoplasms per 100,000 of same age, female, 1960-1964, Berlin, capital of G.D.R.

	I.C.D.	Age groups (5-year classes)																	
	No.	0-	5-	10-	15-	20-	25-	30-	35-	40-	45-	50-	55-	60-	65-	70-	75-	80-	All
Lip	140					0.4				0.7			0.4	0.8	1.4	0.6	1.7	2.4	0.4
Tongue	141										1.7	0.4	1.1	0.4	0.9	2.8	1.7	3.5	0.7
Salivary glands	142					0.9	0.5	0.6	1.3	1.4	0.6		1.9	3.3	2.3	1.1	1.7	3.5	1.1
Mouth	143-145											0.4		0.4	1.4	1.1		1.2	0.3
Pharynx	146-149								0.7	2.7	0.6	0.4	1.1	3.2	2.7	2.9	3.5	1.2	1.2
Mesophagus	150								0.7	0.7		0.4	1.9	0.8	4.6	9.1	16.5	14.1	2.2
Stomach	151					0.4	0.5	2.5	5.9	9.5	14.2	20.9	33.0	57.9	77.0	114.3	118.7	70.7	29.8
Small intestine	152					0.4	0.5				0.6	0.4		1.6	1.8	1.1		1.2	0.5
Colon	153			0.8		0.4		0.6	2.0	2.0	6.2	12.2	21.1	26.9	47.3	59.7	59.8	45.9	16.2
Rectum	154					0.4	0.5		1.3	3.4	4.5	12.2	18.5	28.6	37.8	36.4	40.7	30.6	12.8
Liver	155							0.6		1.4	1.1	3.0	3.7	3.7	2.7	6.8	6.9	7.1	2.1
Gall bladder	156									1.4	5.1	6.5	10.0	19.6	34.6	40.4	45.1	44.8	11.2
Pancreas	157										1.1	3.8	7.4	11.0	14.1	15.3	21.7	9.4	4.9
Other digestive organs	158-159								0.7	0.7	1.7	1.1	2.2	2.9	2.3	4.0	2.6	1.2	1.2
Nose, Sinuses	160				1.4						0.6	0.8	1.1	0.4	1.8	1.7	3.5	2.4	0.7
Larynx	161								2.6	0.7	0.6	2.3	1.1	1.6	1.4	0.6	0.9		0.8
Trachea, Bronchus	162					0.9	0.5		2.0	3.4	9.1	11.4	25.2	24.1	21.4	17.6	20.8	13.0	9.8
Pleura	163.0							0.6	0.6						0.9	1.1	1.7	1.2	0.3
Mediastinum	163.1									1.4	0.6	0.4	0.7	1.6		1.1	0.9	1.2	0.5
Bone	170				0.7	0.9	0.5	1.9	0.7	0.7	0.6	0.8	0.7	2.4	1.4	4.5	4.3	1.2	1.2
Connective tissue	171				0.7	0.9				0.7	1.7	2.7	0.7	0.9	1.8	4.0	0.9	3.5	1.1
Melanoma, Skin	172,173	0.6			1.4	3.5	4.0	8.1	16.4	12.2	28.3	31.2	32.6	54.3	86.5	107.5	130.8	155.5	35.9
Breast	174						4.0	9.4	31.4	69.8	107.7	87.8	92.0	104.0	128.9	122.2	142.1	127.2	61.5
Cervix uteri	180	0.6				4.4	22.6	71.8	108.7	156.6	128.1	101.5	80.8	74.6	69.2	56.3	46.8	28.3	58.9
Chorionepithelioma	181					0.4	0.5						0.4						0.1
Corpus uteri	182							0.6	2.0	8.1	18.1	38.8	36.0	39.2	35.0	30.7	35.5	20.0	17.5
Ovary	183	0.6			1.4	1.3	4.5	1.9	6.5	18.3	24.9	34.6	36.0	33.9	42.4	44.9	21.7	16.5	19.1
Vagina, Vulva	184						0.5	1.2	2.6	1.4	4.0	5.3	7.0	11.0	15.5	15.9	19.9	18.8	5.8
Urinary bladder	188										1.7	5.3	5.2	8.2	6.8	9.7	8.7	14.1	3.5
Kidney	189	1.7	0.7			0.4					2.8	6.5	4.5	9.0	9.6	11.4	8.7	5.9	3.8
Eye	190	1.1		0.8						1.4	1.1	2.3	2.6	1.6	1.4	5.1	2.6	3.5	1.4
Brain	191	2.2	0.7	2.4	1.4	1.8	2.5	3.1	2.6	5.4	4.5	7.6	7.0	5.3	3.6	3.4	8.7	7.1	4.1
Nervous system	192			0.8		0.9							0.7	1.6	0.5				0.3
Thyroid	193						0.5	0.6				1.1	1.9	3.7	4.6	2.3	3.5		1.2
Other endocr. glands	194						0.5	1.2	0.7	0.7	1.1	0.8	1.1	1.2	0.5			1.2	0.6
Other localization	195-199					0.4			0.7	1.4	1.7	3.0	6.4	7.7	10.1	13.6	12.1	7.1	3.8
Lympho-a ret. sarcoma	200					0.9		0.6	2.6	1.4	2.3	1.5	1.1	5.3	5.9	7.4	10.4	5.9	2.5
Lymphogranulomatosis	201		1.4	1.6	2.8	4.0	2.0	1.2	3.9	2.7	1.1	1.5	1.9	2.9	3.6	2.3	0.9		2.1
Other lymph. tumors	202				1.4	0.4	0.5	0.6	1.3	1.4	0.6	1.1	0.4	2.0	3.2	1.7		2.4	1.0
Multiple myeloma	203									1.4	1.1	0.8	2.6	4.5	2.3	4.0	3.5		1.3
Acute lymph. leukemia	204.0			0.8		0.4	1.0				0.6	1.1	1.5	0.8	2.3	1.1	2.6		0.8
Chron. lymph. leukemia	204.1						0.5		0.7		1.1	1.9	2.2	4.1	4.1	5.7	6.1	2.4	1.7
Acute myel. leukemia	205.0		1.4			1.3	1.5	1.9	0.7			0.4	1.1	1.6	0.9	1.1	2.6	1.2	0.9
Chron. myel. leukemia	205.1					0.4			0.7	2.7	1.1	1.1	1.9	2.0	3.2	1.7	2.6	2.4	1.2

Table 2 b. Incidence of malignant neoplasms per 100,000 of same age, female, 1965-1969, Berlin, capital of G.D.R.

	I.C.D. No.	Age groups (5-year classes)																	
		0-	5-	10-	15-	20-	25-	30-	35-	40-	45-	50-	55-	60-	65-	70-	75-	80-	All
Lip	140											1.2	0.4		0.5	0.6	0.8	2.1	0.3
Tongue	141								0.6		0.7		0.4	1.3	2.0	2.4	0.8	4.3	0.6
Salivary glands	142				0.8	1.2	0.4	1.0	3.0	2.6	6.9	3.5	2.0	3.3	2.5	2.4	4.2	4.3	2.1
Mouth	143-145				0.8		0.4	0.5			1.3			0.4	1.4	1.2		3.2	0.4
Pharynx	146-149						0.4			0.6	0.7	1.7	3.2	1.2	4.9	3.6	6.7	4.2	1.5
Mesophagus	150									0.6		1.2	2.4	3.3	7.0	8.4	11.0	12.8	2.3
Stomach	151					0.6	1.6	2.4	4.9	5.2	15.8	18.1	37.0	53.0	89.0	128.6	210.1	219.1	38.0
Small intestine	152											0.6	0.4	1.7	1.5	3.0	4.2	3.2	0.7
Colon	153			0.7	0.8	2.9		1.4	5.5	9.1	11.7	15.8	29.8	29.6	70.5	94.3	101.2	127.6	25.2
Rectum	154						0.4	1.0	3.0	7.8	16.5	17.6	27.3	30.9	47.7	67.3	75.1	52.1	18.6
Liver	155						0.4	0.5		1.9	4.1	4.1	4.0	6.7	12.4	15.6	15.2	19.1	4.3
Gall bladder	156								1.8	5.2	2.1	9.4	20.1	32.5	53.6	88.9	100.5	124.4	21.9
Pancreas	157										2.1	8.2	18.1	16.3	27.8	40.2	34.6	42.5	10.1
Other digestive organs	158-159						0.4	0.5	0.6		0.7	2.9	0.8	1.7	2.5	3.6	4.2	3.2	1.1
Nose, Sinuses	160									0.6	0.7	1.8	1.6	1.7	2.0	3.6		5.3	0.9
Larynx	161							0.5		0.6		1.8	1.2	2.9	3.0	0.6	1.7	1.1	0.8
Trachea, Bronchus	162						0.4		1.8	6.5	7.6	19.3	26.6	44.2	66.0	59.5	43.9	30.8	18.0
Pleura	163.0								0.6			1.8	1.6	2.9	1.0	3.0	1.7		0.8
Mediastinum	163.1						0.4			0.6		1.2			1.0	0.6	0.8	3.2	0.4
Bone	170	2.4		2.0	2.3	1.7	1.6		1.8	0.6	1.4	1.8	1.6	0.4	4.0	4.2	8.4	2.1	2.0
Connective tissue	171		0.5			0.6	0.8	1.9	1.8	1.9	1.4	1.2		1.7	2.0	3.6	2.5		1.2
Melanoma, Skin	172,173	0.5	1.1	1.3	0.8	4.0	5.3	7.1	10.3	20.7	34.3	48.0	50.7	65.5	90.4	136.4	145.1	174.4	41.4
Breast	174					0.6	6.9	9.5	37.0	60.3	105.0	102.4	120.7	131.0	139.0	169.4	149.3	149.9	67.2
Cervix uteri	180				0.8	8.7	31.1	75.7	122.5	145.9	142.8	124.1	90.1	76.3	76.0	67.3	43.9	38.3	61.6
Chorionepithelioma	181				1.5		0.4												0.1
Corpus uteri	182					0.6	1.6	1.0	4.2	12.3	28.1	54.4	45.4	45.0	46.7	52.3	44.7	26.6	21.4
Ovary	183			2.0	1.5	5.8	3.3	6.7	15.2	22.7	33.6	40.4	49.5	57.6	53.6	54.7	64.1	53.2	26.5
Vagina, Vulva	184						0.4	1.0	3.0	3.9	4.8	8.2	6.4	8.8	15.9	18.0	26.2	21.3	6.1
Urinary bladder	188								0.6	1.3	2.7	5.3	8.4	10.4	23.8	19.8	17.7	30.8	6.4
Kidney	189	0.5	0.5					1.9	3.0	1.9	5.5	7.6	11.3	13.3	15.4	13.2	37.1	20.2	7.0
Eye	190	1.9								0.6	0.7	3.5	2.8	0.8	2.5	1.2	3.4		1.1
Brain	191	1.9	2.1	0.7	1.5	3.5	3.3	1.9	6.1	5.8	4.8	12.9	10.5	10.4	12.9	19.2	13.5	24.5	7.4
Nervous system	192		0.5				0.8			1.9		0.6	2.4	1.3	0.5	0.6		1.1	0.6
Thyroid	193					0.6		0.5	1.3		1.4	2.9	2.4	3.8	4.0	10.2	5.1	3.2	2.0
Other endocr. glands	194	1.4	0.5				0.8	1.4	0.6			0.6	2.0	2.1	1.5			4.3	0.9
Other localization	195-199						0.4			0.6	4.1	3.5	8.8	10.4	11.9	15.6	14.3	11.7	4.6
Lympho-a ret. sarcoma	200	0.5	0.5	0.7		0.6	0.4		0.6	1.3	1.4	2.9	2.4	5.4	7.9	9.6	15.2	4.3	2.9
Lymphogranulomatosis	201	1.0		0.7	2.3	2.3	2.0	3.3	0.6	2.6	0.7	1.8	4.4	2.5	3.0	5.4	9.3	3.2	2.5
Other lymph. tumors	202						0.4		0.6	0.6	0.7		0.8	0.8	1.5	2.4	0.8	2.1	0.6
Multiple myeloma	203					0.6				1.3	0.7	2.3	4.0	5.8	3.0	6.0	10.1	5.3	2.2
Acute lymph. leukemia	204.0	1.9	0.5	2.0		0.6			0.6	1.9	1.4	1.8	2.8	1.7	4.5	4.2	5.9	4.3	1.9
Chron. lymph. leukemia	204.1	0.5								0.6	0.7	1.8	0.4	4.6	5.5	8.4	8.4	6.4	2.0
Acute myel. leukemia	205.0	1.4	1.6			0.6	0.4	0.5	0.6		1.4	0.6	1.2	1.3	3.5	2.4	5.1	3.2	1.3
Chron. myel. leukemia	205.1	1.0	0.5		0.8		0.4	1.0	1.2	1.3	1.4	1.8	2.4	1.3	2.5	1.8	1.7	2.1	1.2
Acute leukemia	207.0														0.5				0.03
Chron. leukemia	207.1											0.6							0.03

Table 3. Cancer of selected sites. Age-adjusted mortality ratio in the regions of the G.D.R., 1960-1969. Mortality for the G.D.R. is set as 100

Region	Stomach		Colon		Rectum		Breast		Cervix
	m	f	m	f	m	f	m	f	f
Rostock	103	100	81	85	90	99	68	105	106
Schwerin	104	111	76	85	83	100	112	98	103
Neubrandenburg	105	107	77	79	82	93	93	103	114
Potsdam	91	98	98	86	95	102	112	99	100
Frankfurt	94	98	107	87	102	82	116	94	106
Cottbus	95	97	83	97	97	88	101	94	95
Magdeburg	94	96	95	96	107	97	77	107	104
Halle	98	98	87	92	101	103	101	99	106
Erfurt	86	85	92	98	105	100	118	96	102
Gera	107	111	113	100	112	120	67	92	92
Suhl	100	100	102	91	108	114	88	86	92
Dresden	99	94	97	97	97	94	120	97	93
Leipzig	106	104	103	104	104	101	87	108	101
Karl-Marx-Stadt	117	116	120	116	100	100	109	93	89
Berlin	87	89	132	132	103	105	116	118	109
DDR (= 100)	71	37	13	13	17	11	0.5	23	27

As can be seen, death rates for gastric cancer are lower in Berlin than in the other regions, while the mortality of cancer of the colon, cervix uteri, and mammary gland is considerably higher than in some other regions. The differences in mortality are consistent with regional morbidity differences reported earlier.

Since the population of the G. D. R. is ethnically homogeneous, except for the small minority group of the Sorbs, it can be concluded from the study that in the main environmental conditions are responsible for the differences in cancer risk. The situation in Berlin is consistent with that in other strongly urbanized and industrialized areas. High incidence and mortality for cancer of the breast and colon is reported, for instance, from Great Britain, where the ratio of breast to cervical cancer is exactly the reverse: in places where the mortality of breast cancer is high, that of cancer of the cervix is low and vice versa, so that the sum of the two is approximately constant (5). In the G. D. R. we find the highest mortality for both localizations in Berlin.

This brief review of regional differences is also intended to show the necessity of exact epidemiological studies aimed at the recognition and elimination of carcinogenic factors, which would be helpful in the institution of regional schemes for cancer control.

Analysis of the Quality of Medical Care

As the registration forms are similar to a concise case history record, they allow evaluation of progress in cancer control, and thus provide information about the quality of medical care. Analysis of cancer reports from a whole county or region has the big advantage over clinical reports that there is no distortion as a result of selection and it is possible to determine the average state of cancer detection and cancer treatment. The situation, of course, is less favorable, on the whole, than could be anticipated on the basis of clinical statistical reports, which are frequently issued by specialized and university institutions and whose basic purpose is to give evidence of progress.

In Berlin we have analyzed the average state of detection and treatment for a number of frequent carcinomas, and we again refer to carcinoma of the cervix as an example.

For each of the two five-year periods 1960-64 and 1965-69, a little over 1,600 cases of invasive carcinoma of the cervix were reported. Stage distribution was little altered, except that the proportion of stage I rose from about 45 percent to 49 percent, but the sum of the almost incurable stages III and IV remained constant. We now have the 5-year survival rates for the years 1960-64 and 1965. As anticipated, they are lower than those contained in the biggest publication containing clinical statistics, the "Annual Report." In the second period, there was a tendency towards a more aggressive operative treatment while the use of irradiation therapy alone was less frequent. According to the stage distribution we can expect that the mortality for 1965-69 will be the same as for the preceding period. If it should be markedly lower, this might be due to a change in therapeutic approach. We realize, of course, that the value of competing therapeutic methods can never be judged from regional statistics. However, they are valuable for this purpose too, providing preliminary information that can be used to improve the planning of prospective trials. We therefore prepared a controlled clinical trial in 1972, in which several Berlin hospitals are taking part and which is aimed at finding out whether operative treatment alone or surgery in combination with radiotherapy is the more effective approach.

In the period from 1960 to 1964, no more than 240 patients with carcinoma <u>in situ</u> of the cervix uteri were registered, as against 640 in 1965-69. The returns for 1970 and 1971 reveal a further increase in registered precanceroses and a shift of relation from stage 0 to the invasive stages, reflecting increased activity in early recognition of cervical carcinoma. However, since 640 preinvasive forms compare with more than 1,600 invasive forms, it is clear that the efforts made at that time were inadequate. The necessary steps have since been taken towards a radical improvement of the early recognition of cancer of the cervix. Thus, cytological laboratories in Berlin will be expanded between 1972 and 1975 to allow every woman between 20 and 60 years of age to have a prophylactic examination at biannual intervals. The number of women examined rose from 22,000 in 1971 to more than 50,000 in 1972, and to 110,000 in 1973, and more than 600 cases of carcinoma in situ were detected by cytological screening. In 1975 it will be possible to examine 330,000 women. The cancer registry allows a check on the effectiveness of such a scheme and the implementation of appropriate steps.

The incidence of cancer in the G. D. R. is about 320 per 100,000 at present, but is considerably higher, almost 500, in Berlin. This is not only due to the higher percentage of elderly people in Berlin compared with the rest of the country (about 20 percent of the population are retiring age or over, i.e. men from the age of 65 onward, and women from 60 years onward), but also to the fact that in Berlin the population of people dying in hospital is greater than in rural areas,and consequently the necropsy rate is higher. In new cases, tumors diagnosed after death are also counted, and these amount to more than 10 percent of all tumors registered in Berlin. For carcinoma of the colon the corresponding figure is approximately 15 percent and the figure is even higher for lung carcinoma. These data also provide information on how management of cancer can be improved.

As a result of the analyses mentioned above, efforts are currently being made to concentrate the treatment of malignant tumors in efficient clinical institutions over the next few years, because diagnosis and therapy of cancer involves fairly high technical expenses, e.g. irradiation equipment, close contact between specialists of several medical disciplines, proximity of a histological laboratory and, of course, highly qualified personnel. We therefore expect better results from the concentration of medical services. The cancer registry will be helpful in providing a constant check on the efficiency of these measures.

Thus the cancer registry in the G. D. R. is being used in various ways as an administrative means for planning and directing cancer control and for immediate medical and social care of cancer patients. It must be mentioned finally that we are making efforts to rationalize the operation of the cancer registry, because our current methods are essentially the same as were introduced in 1952. We now have to consider how to make use of modern technology to reduce expenditure, to improve evaluation and to render the cancer registry more effective in the organization of measures for the management of cancer.

References

1. Das Berliner Gesunheitswesen. Bericht über die Entwicklung des Gesundheitswesens in der Hauptstadt der DDR, Berlin 1972. Büro für Sozialhygiene des Magistrats von Groß-Berlin 1972.

2. BERNDT, H., WILDNER, G. P., KLEIN, K.: Regional and social differences in cancer incidence of the digestive tract in the German Democratic Republic. Neoplasma 15, 501 (1968).
3. BERNDT, H., WILDNER, G. P.: Veränderungen der Krebsmorbidität in der DDR 1956-1966. In: Fortschritte der Krebsforschung in den sozialistischen Ländern. Referate und Vorträge des 2. Internationalen Berliner Krebssymposiums, November 1969 in Berlin-Buch. p. 221. Dresden: Steinkopff 1971.
4. Das Gesundheitswesen der Deutschen Demokratischen Republik 1971. 6th yearly volume. Berlin: Akademie für Ärztliche Fortbildung der DDR 1971.
5. STOCKS, P.: Breast cancer anomalies. Brit. J. Cancer 24, 633 (1970).

Linkage of the Icelandic Cancer Registry to an Icelandic Population File

O. Bjarnason and M. Magnusson

1. Introduction

The first settlers of Iceland are believed to have come to the country from Norway in the later part of the ninth century. In the Book of the Settlement, written about 1130, more than four hundred settlers are mentioned by name, the majority of whom were of Norwegian origin. Although the language of the Norwegian Vikings prevailed in the country, recent blood group and anthropological studies seem to indicate that the Scottish and Irish element among the settlers may have been larger than previously assumed (6, 3, 2). The main routes taken by the settlers are shown in Fig. 1.

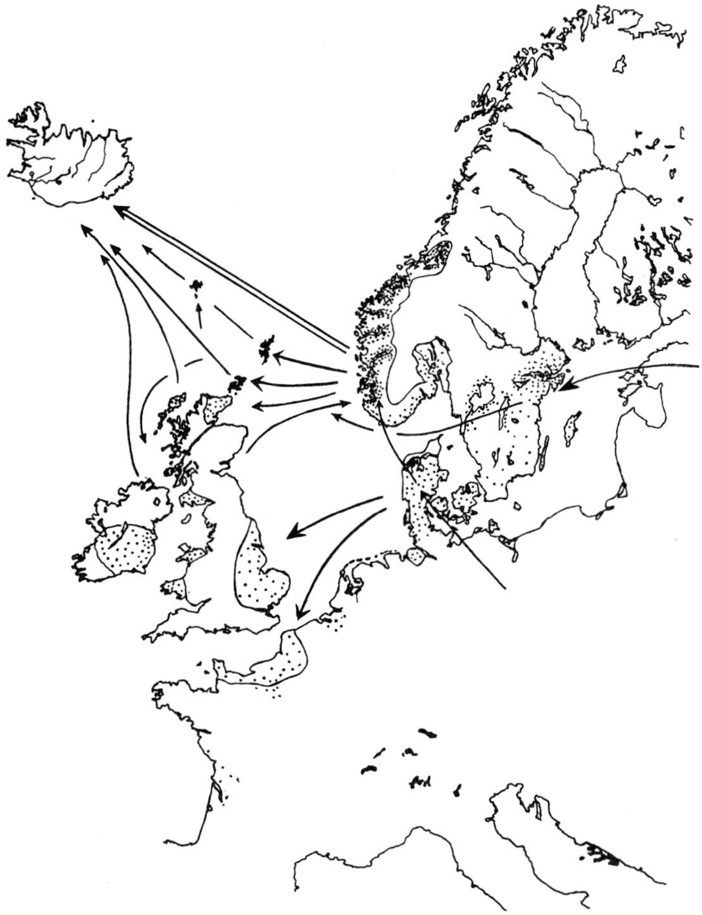

Fig. 1. Main routes taken by settlers of Iceland

The country is thought to have been fully settled in some 60 years, i.e. all inhabitable land had been occupied although the inhabitants and their homesteads increased in numbers as time went by (4). It may even be assumed that the population increased steadily until about 1200; the number of inhabitants at this time has been calculated as 78,000 (7). A curve has been drawn by Steffensen to show the changes in the Icelandic population from the early settlement until 1960 (Fig. 2).

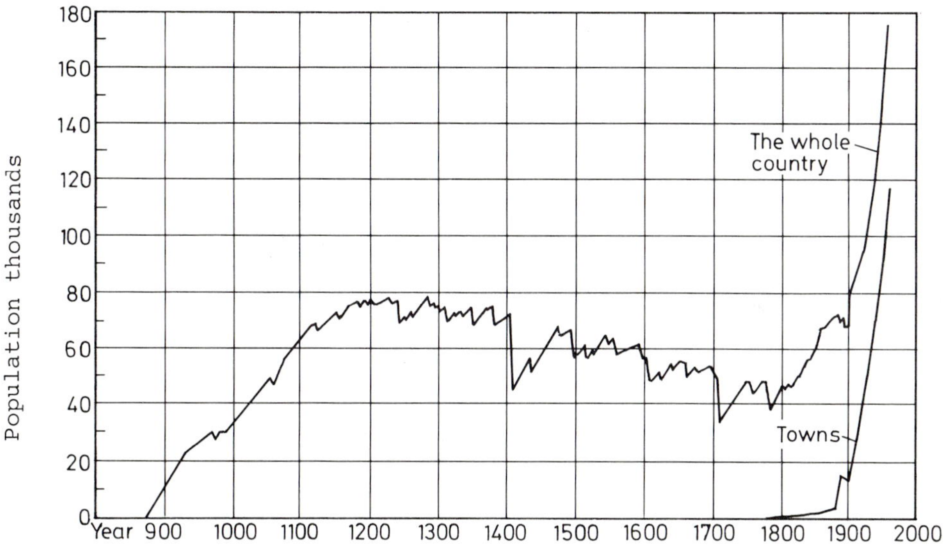

Fig. 2. Population of Iceland 874 - 1960

The struggle with the hardships of life on the island, such as frequent epidemics, natural disasters, and famines resulted in a decline of the population from about 1400 until the early years of the 19th century. Since then the population has been steadily increasing, especially since the beginning of the 20th century, reaching the 200,000 mark in 1968. The lowest point was reached after an epidemic of variola in 1707 when the population sank below 40,000.

It should be mentioned here that one of the first censuses covering a whole nation was performed in Iceland in 1703. In this census every individual living in the country is noted by name, occupation, age and place of residence. From that time onwards accurate data on changes in the population are on record.

Immigration into Iceland has been negligible from the settlement until the present day. Emigration of people from Iceland has not had any influence except in the later years of the 19th century when a number of people moved over to North America.

2. The Icelandic Population File

The Genetics Committee of the University of Iceland has been working for some years on a project in human genetics. Iceland is particularly suitable for such a project for several reasons. The population is relatively small, at present just above 200,000, and the number of Icelanders alive in 1910 and of those born since is less than 300,000. This is a manageable number even for small or medium-sized computers. Demographic records are available in fairly good form from 1916, and records of births, deaths and marriages are available in parish registers back to 1816. In 1952 a National Register was set up containing all individuals living in Iceland. This is updated annually. Extensive genealogical data are available in books and publications.

The computer side of this project has largely been concerned with linking the various records available. The aim of this work is to build up a Genealogical File for the purpose of generating pedigrees by computer and finding family relationship. The basic element in this file concerns the birth event with information on the child-father-mother triplet, which is derived from the birth records. The work now in progress is concerned with establishing a genealogical file of Icelanders who were alive in December 1910 and appear in the census that year and of those who have been born since that time. When this file is in good shape it should be easy to trace families backwards, e.g. finding the father of a child in its birth records and then finding the father's birth record where his parents are found, etc. Finally, a file of individuals starting with each person's birth and ending eventually with his death and containing various types of information such as blood group, medical history, cause of death, may be set up.

2.1. Records

Most of the records have been obtained from the Statistical Bureau of Iceland, which has been extremely cooperative. Without its full cooperation the project would never have been started. All the records that will be discussed have been punched on cards. The number of cards is now about 650,000.

2.2. Birth Records

The birth record cards from 1916 onwards are punched from the records kept at the Statistical Bureau. For the period 1916-1966 there are about 170,000 cards. The information contained in these cards is as follows:

1. Date of birth
2. First and second name of child (first three letters of each name).
3. Sex
4. First name and surname of father (first three letters). Normally the surname of the child is derived from the frist name of the father (patronym).
5. Date of birth of father or his age (in older records).
6. First name and surmane of the mother. In most cases the surname of the mother is derived from the first name of her father but is not the same as the surname of the husband.
7. Date of birth of mother or her age (older records).
8. Place of birth (4-digit code).
9. Single or multiple birth.
10. Legitimate or illegitimate birth.
11. Live birth or stillbirth.

It is, of course, crucial to establish the identity of the child uniquely, i.e. to link the birth record to the National Register, if the individual is alive, or to the death records, if he, or she, is dead. The aim is to establish almost complete linkage of these records for those born from 1916 onwards.

2.3. The National Register

The register, which was first established in 1952, covers all living individuals in Iceland on 1st December each year. There are now records of about 200,000 persons in the register. Great care is taken to ensure that the information is correct and complete, for the register forms the basis for other registers, such as the voting register, income tax register, social security register, and health service register. One punched card contains the following information pertaining to each individual:

1. Name.
2. Date of birth, year (last two digits), month, day.
3. Birth number, which is a 2-digit number distinguishing the individuals born on the same day.
4. Place of birth.
5. Sex.
6. Marital status.
7. Nationality.
8. Religion.
9. Place of residence.
10. Occupation.
11. Name identification number.

The date of birth and the birth number give an 8-digit number which identifies the individual uniquely, e.g. 26101935. Apart from giving unique identification this number thus contains valuable information, the date of birth. This number is the most important single item of information in our files. The essential purpose of linking the birth records to the National Register is to transfer this number for the child into its birth record. When these 8-digit numbers have been obtained for the triplet in the birth records (child-father-mother) we need only 24 digits to identify uniquely these three persons and give their dates of birth. Note that the National Register does not contain information about the parents, apart from the first name of the father in most cases, and cannot therefore form the basis of a genealogical file. Since the National Register only contains records of living persons we must go to the death records for those who have died.

2.4. Death Records

Death certificates are available in the Statistical Bureau from 1916. Prior to that deaths were recorded in parish registers or church books. The number of death records which have been punched for the period 1916-1966 is about 63,000. One punchcard contains the following information on the deceased:

1. Date of death.
2. Cause of death (WHO code).
3. Name (6 letters of the first name and the surname).
4. Sex.
5. Date at birth (prior to 1940 the age of death only is recorded in the majority of cases).
6. Place of birth (not known in most cases).
7. Name of the mother if child died unbaptized.
8. Legitimate or illegitimate birth if infant death.

9. Marital status of deceased.
10. Occupation.
11. Place of residence.

For unique identification a 2-digit number outside the range of numbers used by the Statistical Bureau for the National Register is added to the date of birth. On linkage to a birth record this is transferred to that record giving an 8-digit identification number corresponding to the 8-digit number in the National Register for living persons. The date of death and cause of death are also transferred to the birth record.

Death records for the period December 1st 1910 till December 31st 1915 have been obtained from parish registers and punched in the same form as those from 1916 onwards. These cards number just over 6,000.

2.5. Marriage Records

The marriage records for the period 1916-1964, just over 45,000 records, have been punched on cards from documents in the Statistical Bureau. The records for the period 1911-1915, just under 3,000, have been obtained from the parish registers and punched on cards in the same form. The information contained in these cards is as follows:

1. Date of marriage.
2. Place of marriage.
3. First name, middle name and surname of bridegroom (first 6 letters of each).
4. Name of bride, in same form as 3.
5. Marital status of bridegroom prior to this marriage.
6. Place of birth of bridegroom.
7. Date of birth of bridegroom.
8. Nationality of bridegroom.
9. Marital status of bride prior to this marriage.
10. Place of birth of bride.
11. Date of birth of bride.
12. Nationality of bride.
13. Consanguinity.

The consanguineous marriages are of particular interest for human genetics. For the period 1916-1964 650 are recorded, and of these 379 are between first cousins. Quite apart from their intrinsic interest the marriage records are of great value for filling in the dates of birth of parents on birth records where this information is missing.

2.6. The 1910 Census

For the period before 1916, records of births marriages and deaths are available only in parish registers. Since these are neither complete nor accurate it was decided to base further work on the census of December 1st 1910. The number of records in the census is about 90,000, but of these 4000 - 5000 are duplicates, since the actual population at that time was just over 85,000. Of course the census does not contain complete information on parentage, but this will gradually be complemented with data from parish registers and other sources. The census of 1910 and the birth records of those born from 1911 contain records of 280,000 Icelanders, 200,000 of whom are alive today. The number of generations in this file will be 4 - 6. It will therefore provide a good and manageable set of data for genetic purposes.

The principal items of information in the census cards are as follows:

1. Date of birth, or age.
2. Sex.
3. Place of birth.
4. Marital status.
5. Year of marriage.
6. Name.
7. Number of children, alive and dead, on Dec. 1, 1910.
8. House identification number.
9. Position of person in household, e.g. son of head of household.

2.7. Blood Group Records

Data on the blood group of donors, recipients and mothers (prenatal blood) have been collected and filed at the Blood Bank in Reykjavik since 1953. The data available in August 1965 were punched on cards with the permission of the Blood Bank. The approximate number of cards is as follows:

Donors	12,000 cards
Recipients	12,000 cards
Mothers	16,000 cards
	40,000 cards

Duplications occur both between groups and to a lesser extent within groups. The distribution of the ABO blood groups in this material was found to be as follows: group O, 14972 individuals, group A, 8586 individuals, group B, 2909 individuals and group AB, 661 individuals.

3. The Cancer Registry

The Icelandic Cancer Registry is under the auspices of the Icelandic Cancer Society and was established in early 1954. The Registry covers the whole of the country and the organization has been described elsewhere (1). The material is collected from three main sources. Firstly all patients entering hospitals in the different parts of Iceland with an initial diagnosis of cancer are reported to the Registry. Secondly all histopathologically registered cases and cases confirmed at post-mortem examination are registered. Lastly, the Statistical Bureau of Iceland permits access to all the death certificates issued each year. By this means it is believed that practically all cases diagnosed as cancer are registered.

3.1. Some Trends in Cancer Incidence

In previous publications (5) it has been shown that the three most common forms of cancer in men in Iceland are carcinoma of the stomach, prostata and lung. Carcinoma of the stomach being by far the most frequent, accounting for approximately one-third of all cases of cancer in men. In women the three most common forms are carcinoma of the breast, stomach and uterine cervix. The percentage contribution to the total number of cases in each sex of the 10 most frequent cancer sites in Iceland is shown in the table below.

Percentage contribution to the total in each sex of the 10 most frequent cancer sites in Iceland

Males		Females	
Stomach	30.4	Breast	21.7
Prostate	9.8	Stomach	13.3
Lung	6.7	Cervix	9.8
Colon	5.1	Ovary	5.8
Kidney	4.8	Corpus uteri	5.7
Nervous system	4.5	Colon	5.3
Leukemia	4.1	Thyroid	3.8
Mal. lymph.	3.5	Nervous system	3.8
Pancreas	3.5	Lung	3.3
Lip.	3.4	Kidney	3.1

In the eighteen years since the establishment of the Icelandic Cancer Registry there have been some changes in incidence trends of a number of cancer forms. The most conspicuous of these changes have been the downward trend in the incidence of carcinoma of stomach (1), and a corresponding upward trend (although numerically not as high) in the incidence of carcinoma of the large bowel.

Of special interest is the substantial increase in the incidence of carcinoma of the lung, which has been discussed more thoroughly elsewhere (8). This increase in the number of patients with lung cancer has followed the increase in cigarette consumption in the country in preceding years.

4. Linkage of the Cancer Registry to Blood Group Records and the Population File

One of the aims of the Cancer Registry has been to collect information which might throw some light on genetic influences on cancer incidence and other genetic problems concerning cancer etiology. In order to further this aim, a close collaboration has been set up between the Cancer Registry and the Genetic Committee of the University of Iceland.

The first results of this collaboration have been presented in a paper (2) dealing with the blood groups of the Icelanders and the linking of cases of carcinoma of the stomach and blood groups. The results of the linking of stomach cancer cases and blood groups are shown in the table below.

Blood Groups in Cancer of Stomach

Blood Groups	O	A	B	Relative Risk (A/O)	Relative Risk (B/O)
Cancer Cases Number F+M	169	113	32	1.17	0.97

Another project on cancer genetics is under way in collaboration with the International Agency for Research on Cancer in Lyon. This comprises the linkage of all cases of breast cancer found in the Cancer Registry to the Population File of the Genetics Committee. This will be the first real test of the computerized genealogical file in Iceland.

Acknowledgements

This work has been supported by a grant from the Atomic Energy Commission, Contract No. AT(30-1)-3548.

References

1. BJARNASON, Ó.: Cancer Incidence in Iceland. In: Racial and Geographical Factors in Tumor Incidence. Pfizer Medical Monograph No. 2, 117. Edinburgh: University Press 1967.
2. BJARNASON, Ó., BJARNASON, V., EDWARDS, J. H., FRIDRIKSSON, S., MAGNUSSON, M., MOURANT, A. E., TILLS, D.: The Blood Groups of the Icelanders. Ann. Eugen. (1973).
3. DONEGANI, J. A., DUNGAL, N., IKIN, E. W., MOURANT, A. E.: Blood Groups of Icelanders. Ann. Eugen. 15, 147 (1950).
4. JÓHANNESSON, J.: Íslendinga Saga (The History of the Icelanders), p. 27 and 47. Ísafoldarprentsmiðja: Almenna Bókafélagið 1956
5. RINGERTZ, N., Ed.: Cancer Incidence in Finland, Iceland, Norway and Sweden. Acta path. microbiol. scand. A. Suppl. 224 (1971).
6. STEFFENSEN, J.: Uppruni Íslendinga (The Origin of the Icelanders) In: Samtíð og saga 3. Reykjavik: 1946.
7. STEFFENSEN, J.: Islands folkemængde gennem tiderne. Medsk. Forum, 16, 129 (1963).
8. THORARINSSON, H., HALLGRÍMSSON, J., BJARNASON, Ó., PETERSEN, G.: Dis. Chest. 52, 754 (1967).

Experiences of the Cancer Registry in Slovenia

B. Ravnihar and V. Pompe-Kirn

Introduction

This report presents some experiences of the Slovene Cancer Registry, which began operations more than twenty-three years ago. They might be of interest in the development of new registries and for those facing similar problems to those encountered in our Registry. As the history and the operating techniques of our Registry have already been described elsewhere (1 - 6), they will be only briefly touched on here.

Legislation

Country-wide permanent cancer registration was initiated on a voluntary basis in Slovenia in 1949 by the Institute of Oncology in Ljubljana, the only cancer center in the Socialist Republic of Slovenia (situated in the north-western part of Yugoslavia). As the hospitals' response to this incentive was promising, the Slovene Government issued a regulation in 1950, by which cancer was made a notifiable disease in the Republic. By the same regulation "The Cancer Registry of Slovenia" was officially instituted at the Institute of Oncology, Ljubljana and the basic notification procedures were prescribed. Although no sanctions have ever been executed on institutions or individuals for omitting notification, we still feel that in the circumstances in our country compulsory cancer notification is the only way of maintaining registration, as it presents an efficient statutory support for the Registry's requirements.

Facilities

Otherwise the conditions for permanent population-based cancer registration in Slovenia are favorable in many respects. The population that the Registry covers is not too large - according to the data of the census in 1971 it now numbers over 1,718,000, and it is well defined geographically as well as by nationality. The health services are of a relatively high standard. In all there are 32 reporting hospitals, and 17 regional health centers which are obliged to notify any newly diagnosed cancer case that has not been sent to hospital for whatever reason. By our governmental regulation the physicians alone are charged for the issue of death certificates.

Private practice does not exist, and it can be assumed that nearly all patients in whom cancer has been diagnosed or suspected are sent to a hospital as there are no facilities for treating cancer elsewhere.

The Seat of the Registry

The advantage that the Registry is situated in the Institute of Oncology should be especially emphasized. As radiotherapy and chemotherapy services are almost completely concentrated in the Institute, which covers the relevant needs of cancer patients over the whole of the country, sooner or later in the course of their illness about 50 percent of them are admitted to this institution. In addition, it is the only hospital which regularly carries out periodic follow-up examinations of cancer patients who have been treated there. These circumstances no doubt add a great deal to the completeness of the information about the individual cases, and especially of follow-up statements. Furthermore, the Institute's physicians, including pathologists, are always at hand to offer any additional information or interpretation of the data concerning the diagnosis or therapy if necessary.

Purposes

The Registry started with the aim of providing data that were adequate for the needs of the national and regional public health authorities in planning the cancer control program as well as for the purposes of epidemiological and clinical investigations. In setting up operating procedures and designing the record forms, the experience of the Danish Cancer Registry and of the cancer registration in France were used as a guide.
From its inception on the program of our Registry has included the collection not only of incidence but also of follow-up data on the registered cases.

Revision of the System after the First Decade

In 1960, i.e. at the end of the first decade of the Registry's operation, a system of mechanical data processing and tabulation was introduced, as it became evident that the large, and steadily increasing, amount of data compiled by the Registry could no longer be used to full advantage with manual processing alone. On this occasion all operation procedures of the Registry were revised. The experiences of the Connecticut Tumor Registry system were very helpful in this revision. Our new code is based on the Uniform Punch Card Code, which is used by the End Results Evaluation Section of the National Cancer Institute, U.S.A.

All the abstract cards filed up to 1961 were thoroughly reviewed, and the recoded data were transferred to IBM punch cards. For anatomical sites the International Classification of Diseases was introduced at that time. For histological classification the nomenclature and coding recommended by UICC and issued by WHO in 1956 (WHO/HS/CANC/24 Code) has been adopted use in the Registry.

At the time of the revision certain items which had been recorded up to then were omitted. The ones eliminated were those which had proved to be useless for some reason, either because they were usually not available or could not be elicited, or were unreliable or because they were too detailed, e.g. marital status, occupation, onset of symptoms, doses delivered in radiotherapy etc. The record forms have accordingly been simplified as much as possible.

Sources of Information

The main sources of information for our Registry are of course the hospitals, which are obliged to report every cancer patient every time he or she is admitted to an in- or out-patient department, regardless of whether or not the patient has been in another hospital before. The legal regulations make the attending physicians responsible for the notification, i.e. for abstracting the data from the hospital case records. In practice, however, in many instances this is done by the record clerks, with or without the supervision of the attending physician. This practice is encountered more often in the University hospitals than in the regional general hospitals. However, the lay clerks to whom the cancer notification is entrusted are usually sufficiently well trained in medical matters to carry out the task properly. In any case, the Registry receives abstracted cancer information that varies widely in quality, either from the physicians or from the clerks. Therefore it is the duty of our Registry staff to check the reliability and completeness of the information obtained, and to solicit the necessary data not supplied.

Notification of cancer cases seen in the out-patient departments of hospitals or at the regional health centers and not been admitted to a hospital is often neglected. Some such cases are certainly brought to the attention of the Registry through the official death certificates, but it is impossible to estimate how many of them escape registration.

Since 1966, in accordance with the revised governmental regulations on cancer registration and control, the copies of the examination reports of all pathology institutions and histological and cytological laboratories have to be sent to the Registry whenever the diagnosis of a clearly malignant neoplasm or other notifiable neoplasm has been established. These "security measures" have improved the proportion of microscopically verified cases, which has reached an average of about 75 percent of all cases in recent years.

Follow-up Information

Follow-up data on the registered cases is provided partly by the regulation already mentioned, i.e. that every registered cancer patient has to be notified to the Registry again whenever readmitted to hospital, whether to an in- or an out-patient department. If no information on a patient is received from these sources for more than one year, the Registry itself has to make inquiries. Every registered cancer patient has to be followed up until the end of his life. According to the most recent Registry statement not more than about 6 percent of the total number of recorded patients are lost to follow-up within the first five years following diagnosis.

The purpose of collecting follow-up information is not only to keep a check on the end results of the treatment and the survival of the patients, but also to improve and complete the data on individual cases. Information acquired during the further course of the disease quite often changes the previously recorded clinical or even microscopical diagnosis concerning the primary site and type of the neoplasm.

Use of Death Certificates

The Registry staff devote a great deal of effort to finding more exact information about the cases which come to the attention of the Registry for the first time by way of the official death certificates. At present more than one third of these are confirmed cancer cases for which hospital notification has been delayed. Of the rest, about 10 percent turn out on the basis of hospital data not to have had cancer at all. The rest are patients who have died at home, and for whom the death certificate is the only source of data and is sometimes completed by the addition of information elicited from the general practitioner. These cases actually account for about 8 percent of all registered cases and most of them are designated as cancer of one of the digestive organs.

The Registry Staff's Responsibility

The staff of our Registry, then, is not only passively but quite actively engaged in collecting and completing information about individual cancer cases. While searching for additional data to clarify certain recorded information it is necessary to be in permanent contact with the persons responsible for cancer notification in the reporting hospitals and in the regional health centers.

Unfortunately there is a constant shortage of staff in our Registry because of financial restrictions. This is the main reason why our Registry cannot be as efficient as would be desirable in publishing data and analyses. However, with its store of information the Registry offers its services in response to increasingly numerous requests from medical and also paramedical professions, and from students of relevant subjects. The data are most frequently requested as a basis or background for clinical studies, for epidemiological studies and investigations, and also for the purposes of professional and public cancer education. Very often these services require extra data processing and an extra work load of the Registry staff. In this connection, the role of the Registry staff in the education of professional people in the utilization and interpretation of the registered data should be pointed out. The program of the last year of the medical curriculum at our Medical Faculty includes one hour in which students are required to acquaint themselves with the Registry's purposes and operation.

Future Tasks

The second decade of the Slovene Cancer Registry's operation has elapsed, and again the need is felt for a revision of its practices and procedures in order to provide more precisely defined and more up-to-date incidence and follow-up information on cancer of particular sites. In view of these needs and of the given circumstances, the following tasks have been scheduled for our Registry service for the near future:

1) Intensification of personal contacts with the reporting institutions and provision of instructions to medical and paramedical professions directly or indirectly concerned with cancer registration. This includes the following obligations:
   - at least once a year, the executive staff of the Registry should pay a visit to the reporting institutions;
   - seminaries on cancer registration are to be organized at regular intervals.

2) Development of a more detailed descriptive code of items for each site of origin of malignant neoplasm, such as that issued by the End Results Section of the National Cancer Institute, U.S.A. in 1967.
This laborious work has not been started yet as it is hoped that the International Association of Cancer Registries will achieve an agreement between Registries of different countries about the adoption of some common standards in the definition of the particular items recorded.

3) Introduction of a computer to be used for data recording and processing.
This work has already started. Thus we hope that by early 1974 all the programs will be written and all the data collected by the Registry between 1969 and 1972 will be ready for transfer to the computer. Later, it is intended to transfer the material compiled for all the past years in successive stages.

We hope these measures will help our Registry to provide the users with information of a higher quality and within a more reasonable time-span. The use of the computer will also make it possible to add more detailed information about the individual cases to the compiled data, as well as to provide more detailed and complete reports on the incidence and survival of cancer cases according to the particular sites.

References

1. RAVNIHAR, B., GRUDEN, I.: Statističen pregled in kratka analiza prijavljenih rakavih obolenj iz področja LRS za leto 1950. Zdr. Vest. 20, 11, 264 (1951).
2. RAVNIHAR, B., VALENTIN, A., BOŽIČ, T., DOIČ, I. and PEČIRER, D.: Cancer in Slovenia, 1955, 6th Annual Statistical Report. Ljubljana: Oncological Institute 1957.
3. RAVNIHAR, B.: Eight years of cancer registration in Slovenia (Yugoslavia). Acta Un. int. Cancr. 16, 1579 (1960).
4. RAVNIHAR, B.: Cancer Incidence in Yugoslavia, Slovenia 1956-1960. In: Cancer Incidence in Five Continents, Volume I. Eds. DOLL, R., PAYNE, P., WATERHOUSE, J.A.H. Geneva: UICC 1966.
5. RAVNIHAR, B.: Cancer Incidence in Yugoslavia, Slovenia 1961-1965. In: Cancer Incidence in Five Continents, Volume II. Eds. DOLL, R., MUIR, C. S., WATERHOUSE, J.A.H. Geneva: UICC 1970.
6. RAVNIHAR, B., Ed.: Rak v Sloveniji - Cancer in Slovenia, Tables (preliminary data) Annual reports for the years: 1965, 1966, 1967, 1968, 1969 and 1970 ("xerox"); Ljubljana: Institute of Oncology.

Cancer Registry Data Versus Mortality Statistics

J. Staszewski

Mortality statistics and cancer morbidity data derived from registration are the two main sources of information on the frequency of cancer occurrence (cancer risk) in developed countries. Other sources, such as hospital or necropsy statistics, are not usually population-based and thus provide heavily biased estimates of cancer risk. Information obtained from cancer surveys is similar to cancer registry data in most of the characteristics discussed below.

As both these types of data, i.e. mortality and morbidity statistics, are often used in studies on cancer epidemiology, it seems worthwhile to compare them as reflections of the true cancer risk and to compare their relative merits and disadvantages.

The criteria on which these comparisons of the value of mortality and morbidity data for estimation of cancer risk will be based are completeness and reliability (the ideal situation would be where all cases were reported and no false positives included), comparability (i.e. with data from other centers), availability of additional information of interest (e.g. on demographic characteristics, histology, other, concomitant diseases, etc.), and cost.

1. Completeness and Reliability

In this respect, both mortality and morbidity statistics depend primarily on the quality of cancer diagnosis in the population under study. False negatives, i.e. cancer cases erroneously diagnosed as other diseases and never recognized as cancers will be missed by a cancer registry and will not be recorded as cancer in mortality statistics. Similarly, false positives usually distort the mortality and morbidity data to an equal degree. Some such false positives, however, may later be correctly diagnosed and a record made that no cancer was present; this may be reflected in either, both, or neither of these kinds of information depending on the prevailing procedures of reporting and registration.

Mortality statistics provide a poor estimate of the occurrence of cancers characterized by a low fatality rate, e.g. skin cancer. Cancer registries, however, are also usually reluctant to claim that their data cover all the skin cancers occurring in their registration area, and sometimes they do not register skin cancer at all.

Interpopulation variation in the treatment and results (due to variation in the availability of treatment, in its quality, in clinical stage distribution, in biologic characteristics bearing on survival, etc.) may distort the estimates of differentials in cancer risk calculated from mortality statistics. However, a comparison of survival rates in six countries (Denmark, England, Finland, France, Norway, United States) showed that variation in treatment policies in the different countries had little bearing on cancer survival and could not account for the observed differences in mortality (6).

Another feature of mortality statistics that can lead to some loss of information is that on the death certificate more than one cause of death is often given, whereas in the routine mortality statistics only one is used (sometimes arbitrarily selected), the one designated the underlying cause. Special studies, however, for example those in the United States, have demonstrated that cancer appears on death certificates as the underlying cause in about 95 percent of cases (5). Therefore, in spite of the omission of a few cancers reported as a contributory cause, not much of the total information on cancer given on death certificates is lost. Rules for the qualification of causes of death, whether underlying or contributory, are laid down by the International Classification of Diseases, Injuries and Causes of Death, whose use is compulsory in most if not all developed countries.

The feature in favor of mortality statistics is that in developed countries each death is reported and is reported only once; in morbidity statistics the same individual is sometimes reported from several sources, creating problems in data processing. Moreover, an individual with cancer may not be reported at all, as shown by the number of cases recorded for the first time on the basis of a death certificate in many cancer registries (4).

2. Comparability

Comparability of data from different regions or time periods is best when the quality is similar and steady. As a rule, this requirement is met better by mortality statistics. The quality of cancer registries' data varies much more than does that of mortality statistics.

Cancer mortality statistics are not very sensitive to such factors as mass surveys, which can cause temporary marked distortions of the incidence data and patterns (9).

The relatively steady level of the quality of mortality data allows more accurate analysis of time trends.

Good mortality statistics are available for the total population of many countries, with a breakdown by important demographic characteristics such as age and sex. This allows meaningful international comparisons in spite of wide differences in the demographic structure of the populations being compared. Comprehensive studies of cancer mortality statistics taking into consideration such characteristics as sex, age, marital status, occupation, socioeconomic class, ethnic derivation, religion, regional differences, and time trends, have been conducted mainly in the United States (e.g. by BURBANK, GLOVER, GORDON et al., HAENSZEL, SEIDMAN), Great Britain (e.g. by ASHLEY, CASE, KENNAWAY, MCKENZIE *et al*., STOCKS), Switzerland (SCHINZ and REICH), Denmark (CLEMMESEN), and Australia (LANCASTER). Mortality statistics compendia have been published by the World Health Organization (7) and by SEGI *et al*. (10, 11, 12, 13). The scope, mode of data presentation, and other important aspects of these publications have since been compared in a review (8).

Information of good quality on cancer morbidity is more limited and is available for smaller populations, in the order of a few millions at most, such as are found in Scandinavian countries, Connecticut state, or selected regions of California state, of Hungary or Poland.

Morbidity data, with some characteristics of the registries producing them, have been listed by DOLL et al. (3, 4). Such statistics are also published by the World Health Organization in their monthly publications. The differences between these publications have been discussed elsewhere (7).

For international comparisons, cancer mortality statistics are often more useful than the available morbidity data. Mortality statistics cover the whole country, as a rule, whereas this is rather the exception with morbidity data, as for the reasons just mentioned, (good) cancer registries usually cover only some selected areas of the country. Selection of these areas and their representativeness for the respective countries varies and is difficult to evaluate. Hence, comparison of morbidity data from, for example, Connecticut and Miyagi cancer registries calls for more reservation when the conclusions are to be extrapolated to the contrasting of the United States and Japan than would be the case if mortality data from these two countries were compared.

3. Availability of Additional Information

The availability of additional information of interest usually enhances the usefulness of cancer morbidity data. The routine mortality statistics provide no details on the location of cancer (e.g. in which part of the stomach), clinical stage, histology, or treatment, whereas such data are usually collected and sometimes published by cancer registries. Data on other, concomitant diseases, in contrast, are more often reported on death certificates than on cancer report cards, but are seldom if ever published.

4. Cost

When the costs, in the broadest meaning of the word, are considered, mortality statistics display a marked superiority over cancer morbidity statistics.

The achievement and maintenance of a good quality of cancer registration requires a great and continuous effort over a long (indefinite) period of time. Furthermore, it usually takes a few years of cancer registration to reach a good and steady quality of morbidity data.

Mortality statistics, on the other hand, are collected routinely (on cancer, and also on all other causes of death). Results are often available in publications or from the unpublished tabulations, but sometimes it may be necessary to prepare special tabulations. Even in such a case, the cost and amount of the work required are very much lower than those incurred by cancer registration.

Registration of cancer morbidity usually provides more complete data on cancer occurrence than is obtainable from mortality statistics, but the difference will not be wide for cancers with a high fatality rate. Furthermore, cancer registration data provide more detailed and precise information, which often makes them especially suitable for sophisticated studies.

On the other hand, mortality statistics are much less expensive, cover more and wider populations (especially of whole countries), are less affected by bias-producing factors and are generally more suitable for broad comparative studies and for time-trend analyses.

The above statements are based on data of a high quality from both sources. In developed countries, mortality statistics are usually reliable and comparable, whereas the quality of cancer registration varies much more widely, which lowers the value of the data for comparative studies. DOLL commented recently that "... in some areas in which cancer registration is incomplete, mortality can provide a better indication of incidence than the official "incidence statistics," particularly for cancer whose fatality is high ..."(2).

When no morbidity statistics are available, cancer incidence can be estimated from mortality data with the aid of conversion factors. Such fators have been published (1, 2).

In spite of all the differences discussed above, information derived from mortality statistics and from morbidity registration is not contradictory, but rather complementary. Experience shows that conclusions based on these two sources of information coincide to a large extent.

From these general considerations we turn to a comparison of the published data derived from cancer registration and mortality statistics covering the same countries.

Cancer incidence rates for 58 populations were published in 1970 in the second volume of "Cancer Incidence in Five Continents" (4). Only nine of these populations, however, are equivalent to whole populations of single countries[1], the rest being populations of selected administrative areas.

Cancer mortality rates for eight of these nine countries (the ninth is the German Democratic Republic) were published about the same time, in 1969, in the fifth volume of "Cancer Mortality for Selected Sites in 24 Countries" (13). Except in the case of Denmark, the periods covered by the data presented in both these publications are similar.

A comparison of the age-adjusted mortality and incidence rates reported from these eight countries will be made for a few selected cancer sites. Selection was based on the availability of data from both sources cited, level of rates (to consider rates based on large numbers which are thus relatively stable), and comparability (liver cancer was therefore omitted).

The malignant neoplasms selected for comparison embrace two cancers with a high fatality rate (stomach and lung cancer), three cancers which are often curable (cancer of intestinal tract, breast, and uterus), and one cancer with a low fatality rate (skin cancer).

From another point of view, out of the six selected cancers two are of superficial location, and are hence usually easy to recognize (especially skin cancer). The other ones, cancers of internal organs, vary in the difficulty of their diagnosis, which is easiest for cancer of the uterus, less easy for gastrointestinal tract cancer, and most difficult for lung cancer.

---

[1]For New Zealand and Israel this is only approximately the case, because in N. Z. the incidence data for Europeans pertain to 91.8 percent of the population (the rest of the population is Maori (6.9 percent), and other races (1.3 percent), whereas in Israel the incidence data pertain to Jews only, i.e. to 88.2 percent of the population of Israel (4).

As shown in Table 1, the difference between the incidence and mortality rates was lowest for stomach and lung cancer, being in the range of 5-22 percent of the incidence rate value in 24 out of 32 comparisons. The negative difference observed for lung cancer in Denmark is easily explained by the rapid increase in the incidence and mortality of lung cancer; incidence data for Denmark pertain to the years 1958-1962 and mortality data to 1964-1965; when mortality rates for 1958-61 (10, 11) are used the difference is a positive one (12 percent for males and 4 for females). The negative differences observed for Scotland seem to indicate incomplete registration of both stomach and lung cancer morbidity.

For intestinal tract cancer the difference between the incidence and mortality rates varies in the range of 24-47 percent,except in Scotland (7 percent for males and 10 percent for females).

For breast cancer this range is 44-69 percent, and for cancer of the uterus it is 46-69 percent. The lowest values of these differences are again those for Scotland. This is consistent with observations in stomach and lung cancer and also in intestinal tract cancer.

For skin cancer the variability of the differences between the incidence and mortality rates is very wide - between 0 and 98.5 percent. In Israel the difference between incidence and mortality rates is negligible, while in Norway it amounts to about half the value of the incidence rate, in New Zealand it is a little higher, and in other countries it is between 78 and 98 percent of the incidence value.

Our findings can be compared with the results of another study (14) which compared the published routine cancer mortality statistics from Israel, (13) with the data recorded by their cancer registry. For each of the sites discussed in the present paper they found that cancer mortality, as reflected in the registry data, was higher than that derived from the routine mortality statistics. However, the differences were not large, usually about 10 percent or less, and would change the rank order of Israel among the 24 countries listed only slightly. The one exception was skin cancer, for which the differences between the two age-adjusted rates were much wider, as were also changes in the rank order.

Our results, and also the study mentioned above (14), indicate that, for the developed countries, the routine mortality statistics give about as good a picture of the distribution of cancer as the morbidity data from good cancer registries and that this is true not only for the cancers that are usually fatal (e.g. lung and stomach cancer), but also for the more curable ones, e.g. of the uterus or breast. Variation in the quality of cancer registration is also apparent; Scotland may be an example of less complete registration.

Data on skin cancer seem to be not very reliable, at least in some of the mortality and morbidity statistics.

This paper should not be seen as an attempt to depreciate the value of cancer registries. I believe that a good cancer registry can produce data of a detail and precision unattainable by the routine mortality statistics, broadening widely the possibilities of epidemiologic research. However, I feel it would be wrong to ask which source of information is superior as a general problem. Both are very useful tools for epidemiologic studies. As with any tool, one of them may be superior in one situation and inferior in another. Moreover, they can be used properly, but they can also be misused, depending on the skill of the investigator and his knowledge of their merits and limitations. Some have been discussed in this paper.

Table 1. Comparison of incidence and mortality data on cancer of selected primary sites in the countries for which data were published both in "Cancer in Five Continents" (4) and by Segi and Kurihara (13)

Country		Stomach (151)		Intestinal tract (152-154)		Lung (162-163)		Breast (170)	Uterus (171-174)	Skin (190-191)	
		Male	Female	Male	Female	Male	Female	Female	Female	Male	Female
Puerto Rico	Mortality[a] 1964-65	27.1	13.2	6.0	5.8	11.0	4.1	6.5	15.2	0.9	0.5
	Incidence[b] 1964-66	28.6	13.7	9.2	10.4	13.6	5.0	20.9	38.2	34.2	34.2
	Difference[c]	1.5	-0.5	3.2	4.6	2.6	0.9	14.4	23.0	33.3	33.7
	Ratio[d]	5.2%	-3.9%	34.8%	44.2%	19.1%	18.0%	68.9%	60.2%	97.4%	98.5%
Israel, all Jews	Mortality[a] 1965-66	18.2	12.6	10.5	10.1	20.8	6.8	21.0	6.2	1.3	1.7
	Incidence[b] 1960-66	25.4	15.4	17.9	18.3	26.4	8.7	44.9	14.8	1.4	1.7
	Difference[c]	7.2	2.8	7.4	8.2	5.6	1.9	20.9	8.6	0.1	0.0
	Ratio[d]	28.3%	18.2%	41.3%	44.8%	21.2%	21.8%	53.2%	58.1%	7.1%	0.0%
Denmark	Mortality[a] 1964-65	21.8	13.4	25.3	20.5	35.8	6.6	23.7	17.6	1.8	2.0
	Incidence[b] 1958-62	27.5	16.4	33.4	28.5	31.4	5.2	44.9	43.1	22.6	15.2
	Difference[c]	5.7	3.0	8.1	8.0	-4.4	-1.4	21.2	25.5	20.8	13.2
	Ratio[d]	20.7%	18.3%	24.3%	28.1%	-14.0%	-26.9%	47.2%	59.2%	92.0%	86.8%
Finland	Mortality[a] 1964-65	39.7	20.4	10.8	10.1	60.7	3.8	13.5	10.4	2.0	1.0
	Incidence[b] 1962-65	44.9	23.4	14.9	14.2	70.0	4.4	29.4	24.8	23.9	20.9
	Difference[c]	5.2	3.0	4.1	4.1	9.3	0.6	15.9	14.4	21.9	19.9
	Ratio[d]	11.6%	12.8%	27.5%	28.9%	13.3%	13.6%	54.1%	58.1%	91.6%	95.2%

Table 1. (continued)

Country		Stomach (151)		Intestinal tract (152-154)		Lung (162-163)		Breast (170)	Uterus (171-174)	Skin (190-191)	
		Male	Female	Male	Female	Male	Female	Female	Female	Male	Female
Norway	Mortality[a] 1964-65	26.0	14.6	13.8	11.5	13.9	2.6	16.9	3.1	2.0	1.5
	Incidence[b] 1964-65	28.8	15.4	19.3	16.7	16.5	3.1	41.0	25.2	3.6	4.0
	Difference[c]	2.8	0.8	5.5	5.2	2.6	0.5	24.1	16.1	1.6	2.5
	Ratio[d]	9.7%	5.2%	28.5%	31.1%	15.8%	16.1%	58.8%	63.9%	44.4%	62.5%
Sweden	Mortality[a] 1964-65	22.0	12.0	16.1	13.5	16.4	3.8	18.5	10.0	1.9	1.3
	Incidence[b] 1962-65	24.8	13.0	25.9	21.6	19.2	4.4	48.6	32.2	8.6	6.1
	Difference[c]	2.8	1.0	9.8	8.1	2.8	0.6	30.1	22.2	6.7	4.8
	Ratio[d]	11.3%	7.7%	37.8%	37.5%	14.6%	13.6%	61.9%	68.9%	77.9%	78.7%
U. K., Scotland	Mortality[a] 1964-65	25.5	14.5	25.1	20.7	75.6	11.4	23.6	10.7	1.8	1.3
	Incidence[b] 1963-66	21.1	10.3	27.1	22.9	67.0	9.9	42.5	20.0	26.4	17.1
	Difference[c]	-4.4	-4.2	2.0	2.2	-8.6	-1.5	18.9	9.3	24.6	15.8
	Ratio[d]	-20.9%	-40.8%	7.4%	9.6%	-12.8%	-15.2%	44.5%	46.5%	93.2%	92.4%
New Zealand: European	Mortality[a] 1964-65	16.5	8.3	21.7	19.0	35.7	4.9	23.3	10.3	3.0	2.3
	Incidence[b] 1962-66	19.1	9.5	41.3	35.2	45.1	6.1	50.2	25.9	6.2	9.1
	Difference[c]	2.6	1.2	19.6	16.2	9.4	1.2	26.9	15.6	3.2	6.8
	Ratio[d]	13.6%	12.6%	47.5%	46.0%	20.8%	19.7%	53.6%	60.2%	51.6%	74.7%

[a] Age-adjusted mortality rate per 100,000 (13) [b] Age-adjusted incidence rate per 100,000 (4)

[c] Difference computed as (incidence - mortality)

[d] Ratio of the difference, defined above, to the incidence rate - expressed as a percentage, and computed as: $\frac{\text{incidence} - \text{mortality}}{\text{incidence}} \cdot 100$

References

1. DOLL, R.: Worldwide distribution of gastrointestinal cancer. Nat. Cancer Inst. Monogr. 25, 174 (1967).
2. DOLL, R.: The geographical distribution of cancer. Brit. J. Cancer 23, 1 (1969).
3. DOLL, R., PAYNE, P., WATERHOUSE, J., Eds.: Cancer Incidence in Five Continents. Geneva: UICC 1966.
4. DOLL, R., MUIR, C. S., WATERHOUSE, J.A.H., Eds.: Cancer Incidence in Five Contients. Vol. II, Geneva: UICC 1970.
5. DORN, H.: Underlying and contributory causes of death. Nat. Cancer Inst. Monogr. 19, 421 (1966).
6. International symposium on end results of cancer therapy. Nat. Cancer Inst. Monogr. 15 (1964).
7. Mortality from malignant neoplasms, 1955-1965. Part I, II. Geneva: WHO 1970.
8. NECTOUX, J., MUIR, C. S.: Cancer morbidity and mortality statistics. Comparison of material published by WHO, Segi and Kurihara and Cancer Incidence in Five Continents. IARC Internal Technical Report 70/006, 1970.
9. PEDERSEN, E.: The presymptomatic diagnosis of cancer: cervix uteri and breast. Proc. roy. Soc. Med., 1189 (1966).
10. SEGI, M., KURIHARA, M.: Cancer Mortality for Selected Sites in 24 Countries. No. 2 (1958-1959). Department of Public Health, Tohoku University School of Medicine, Sendai, Japan, 1962.
11. SEGI, M., KURIHARA, M.: Cancer Mortality for Selected Sites in 24 Countries. No. 3 (1960-1961). Department of Public Health, Tohoku University School of Medicine, Sendai, Japan, 1964.
12. SEGI, M., KURIHARA, M.: Cancer Mortality for Selected Sites in 24 Countries. No. 4 (1962-1963). Department of Public Health, Tohoku University School of Medicine, Sendai, Japan, 1966.
13. SEGI, M., KURIHARA, M.: Cancer Mortality for Selected Sites in 24 Countries. No. 5 (1964-1965). Department of Public Health, Tohoku University School of Medicine, Sendai, Japan, 1969.
14. STEINITZ, R., COSTIN, C.: Cancer mortality. Vital statistics versus cancer registry. Isr. J. Med. Sci. 7, 1405 (1971).

Hints on the Evaluation of a Regional Cancer Registry with no Legal Basis

G. Keding

Cancer is gradually becoming a very serious social and medical problem for nearly all peoples. Our statistical knowledge on cancer does not correspond to the importance of this illness to the society or offer a firm basis for decisions on health policy aimed at helping those whose lives are endangered through cancer. In West Germany there is a wide discrepancy, as far as the statistics available on cancer are concerned, between scientific, well-founded possibilities and methods of practice.

Epidemiological studies on cancer were sponsored in Germany as early as the turn of the century. At that time a program for statistical research work on cancer was drawn up and this is still valid to-day. Even then it was clear that the statistical proceeding relating to causes of death was inadequate. In Hamburg it was realized earlier than elsewhere that careful medical statistics were very important. Parliament and executive showed much interest in this work, and the advantages of Hamburg as a city-state would be well utilized. As suplementary material for evaluation, the Hamburg Cancer Registry (Table 1) compares cases of death (classified according to the organs affected) registered from 1904 to 1918 with those recorded in the period 1954 to 1958.

Table 1. Deaths from Cancer in Hamburg

1904 -	1918	as against	1954 -	1968
7200 ♂	8896 ♀		36018 ♂	34167 ♀
		Distribution by Organ:		
0.0%	0.2%	Brain	1.5%	1.2%
1.4%	0.9%	Skin	0.9%	1.0%
1.5%	0.3%	Mouth	1.3%	0.6%
6.9%	2.2%	Respiratory Tract	32.4%	7.2%
0.1%	11.8%	Mammary Gland	0.1%	15.2%
74.2%	43.8%	Digestive Organs	37.9%	35.7%
43.4%	26.8%	including Stomach	20.0%	15.8%
7.1%	9.3%	Liver & Gallbladder	5.1%	8.8%
3.4%	1.6%	Urinary Tract	7.2%	3.5%
3.1%	28.1%	Genital Organs	9.1%	20.3%
2.3%	1.8%	Others	4.5%	6.5%

The inverse correlation to sex and the shift in the structured figures relevant to involvement of the respiratory tract, the digestive organs and the reproductive organs are notable.

The awakening conscience of society towards cancer patients led to the setting up of special institutions for their care in Hamburg. The City Physician, Professor Sieveking, is considered the initiator of the so-called "Follow-up Patients' Aid Service;" he started this work on 1st January 1929. This was in keeping with the general opinion of the times, that work on the further care of the cancer patients should begin in the hospitals where they were first treated. There was a desire for good team work between hospitals and general practitioners. Nurses took over the care of the patients, their work including the correct supervision of treatment and help prescribed by the doctors.

A record of all important data was kept and up-dated from weekly reports of deaths. The statistical evaluation of these records became an important by-product of the work of the service, which served as the basis for Hamburg's Cancer Registry. The principle of the Registry has remained the same up to the present day.

A lot has been said about the Follow-up Patient's Aid Service. First of all Sieveking published his numerical data, which were later found in publications by different hospital doctors such as HOLTHUSEN and HAMANN, GÖBEL, ABEL, VONESSEN, GAUWERKY, MAASS, SACHS and PAUKA. In 1941 and 1957 a summary of the statistical figures was published by the State Statistical Office of the Free and Hanseatic City of Hamburg, for which we are grateful to this office. The publication can be supplied to anyone interested on request. It is therefore not necessary to go into more detail at this point.

The fight against cancer cannot be won by unrealistic thoughts and wishes. The rather unfortunately limited methods must be applied with the greatest possible efficiency. Epidemiologists and clinical experts can pick out of the Cancer Registry all the important facts needed for the drawing up of policies on health. In Hamburg the emphasis is currently on cancer of the breast; 8329 cases of this condition were registered within 15 years. Fig. 1 shows the classification of the cases, divided into 3-year groups. A shift is evident when the age groups and the percentage of cases are compared. For example, the 50-60-year-olds previously formed the largest group, while now the group of the 60-70-year-olds is the largest. The calculated incidence shows an almost uniform rise in all age groups. This is discussed in more detail in the publication referred to above.

The Hamburg system has hitherto supplied satisfactory statistics on cancer cases. The inception of the State Statistical Office has ensured regular and up-to-date control of the statistics on causes of death. The method covered the proportion of deaths from cancer in cases that could never benefit from after-care. The results indicate that the epidemiology can be recognized without involved legal procedures such as obligatory reporting by doctors.

Science has improved the early diagnosis of different types of cancer. Thus, in 1971, it was possible to introduce cancer screening financed by the health insurances in West Germany. German specialists had been stressing the necessity for these examinations for some decades. We must bear in mind that one consequence of our statistical methods is that less information is recorded in cases of organic cancer that benefit from early diagnosis. The treatment of the early stages of organic cancer does not require so much or such specialized work as cases which are diagnosed later. Cases diagnosed early could thus be treated in small hospitals or in doctors' private clinics. Moreover, because these patients do not need so much social care, there would be less call on our services, in which case much less data would be recorded.

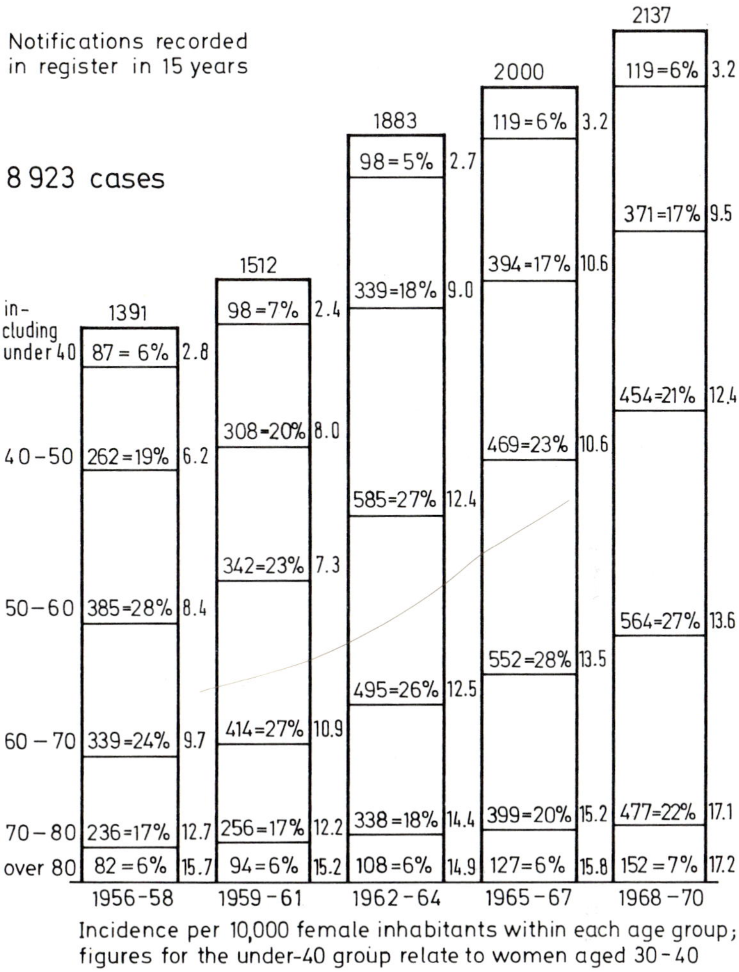

Fig. 1. Cancer of the breast in Hamburg

If statistical records are to continue to be any help at all, and a purposeful fight against cancer is to achieve its aim, all concerned must work together with the Registry.

Medicine is becoming increasingly a social science, and its progress will practically depend on society. It is a pity that epidemiology has not won more recognition as an important field in social medicine. The institution of an up-to-date , workable epidemiological system would involve measures that are not acceptable to the majority of doctors and in fact would not go through our Parliaments. It appears that society is not very well-informed about the facts on this issue.

Doctors seem to be restricted legally, e.g. by the obligatory secrecy that is one of the recognized foundations of our medical practice. Perhaps it would be better to keep epidemiology in the legal field of secrecy in order to give it some sort of impetus. All concerned, particularly the public health service, should think seriously about this problem and try to find the appropriate solution. We doctors could help ourselves and our objectives if we would adopt a more progressive attitude to epidemiology instead of persisting in our present repressive attitude.

Cancer Registry South Württemberg-Hohenzollern. First Report

G. Neumann

1. Introduction

In the Federal Republic of Germany, cancer registries are being kept in Hamburg and in the Saarland. In view of Hamburg's position as a city state and the particular situation of the Saarland, neither of these regions can be regarded as representative of the Federal Republic. Fundamentally, there is a serious demand for more cancer registries in the Federal Republic.

The Württemberg region offered a special opportunity for the establishment of a further cancer registry. A co-operative study of risk groups of carcinoma of the cervix uteri was conducted in 1969-1970, and developed rapidly, effortlessly and quite efficiently into a registry of this type of carcinoma. This established a basis for further efforts in this direction. In the Federal Republic a cancer registry can only be kept on a voluntary basis. A further restriction stems from the professional discretion, which must be respected. Thus, a registry virtually has to be an anonymous basis, which limits it to a descriptive registry of cancer incidence without follow-up.

The decision in favor of a registry was influenced by the following factors:

1) From an overall viewpoint of morbidity statistics, additional models are highly desirable.
2) With rising cure rates for malignomas, the value of death statistics is declining accordingly.
3) The number of factors that mortality statistics cover is rather limited.
4) In the Federal Republic, screening for cancer of the cervix and of the breast has been available to all women over thirty years of age and screening for cancer of the prostate and of the rectum to all men over fortyfive, so that a cancer registry promises additional information relating to the effectiveness of these measures.

This last point was particularly important in the decision reached, because the form of documentation of cancer screening must be supplemented by further data.

Support from the authorities responsible was obtained only for the region South Württemberg-Hohenzollern (which, as of January 1, 1973, comprises the region of Tübingen), a territory with a population of 1,600,000 persons (census 1970), i.e. less than Hamburg but more than the Saarland. All hospitals, pathology and anatomy institutes and dermatologists are requested to participate. In 1971 60 of 110 hospitals participated, and in 1972 73 hospitals. The three pathologists have not reported. This is understandable insofar as only very few of the desired clinical data are at their disposal. If the pathologists did cooperate, then the number of cases reported from two sources would rise considerably, but the completeness of the registry would be improved. Of the 24 dermatologists, 8 cooperated in 1971 and 13 in 1972. The best, almost complete, participation was by the gynecologists. They are followed by the surgeons, while the proportion of internists who responded was appreciably lower. The Landesverband Württemberg zur Erforschung und Bekämpfung des Krebses, the regional anti-cancer association, which keeps the registry, reimburses DM 5.-- for the completion of a questionnaire. The quality of the questionnaires returned varies, but most of the missing data can be elicited by relevant inquiry. Nevertheless, 1.5 percent of the data relating to birth were missing in 1971.

The questionnaire for the cancer registry begun on April 1, 1971 includes:

1. name of reporting hospital or doctor
2. date of birth
3. sex
4. nationality
5. residence
6. date of hospital admission
7. diagnosis
8. stage of malignoma, classified by TNM system or other classification system
9. type of malignoma (carcinoma, sarcoma, etc.)
10. histological findings
11. Mode of verification of diagnosis
12. reasons for diagnosis (symptoms, screening, others)
13. preliminary outcome (discharge, death, still in hospital).

No questions were asked regarding occupation, smoking habits, other possible risk factors, onset of symptoms, the therapy instituted. Each institution that was requested to participate received two forms, one explaining the aims and purposes of the cancer registry, and the other giving additional information of a formal nature and detailed instructions on completion of the computer-readable questionnaire.

The first year, 1971, must be considered as a running-in period and does not permit any real epidemiological statements. Evaluation was therefore carried out in a simplified manner. The problem of double registration was not taken into account, and appropriate correction was planned for 1972.

All institutions taking part in the inquiry were sent a concise report for 1971, and also a set of tables showing the most important results of the total inquiry. Depending on the number of cases, classification was more or less comprehensive and the figures of each reporting unit were also given and explained. No participant took advantage of the offer of additional information. Detailed representation has been given in the annual report of the "Landesverband" for 1972.

2. Results

2.1. Total Number

In Baden-Württemberg in 1971, 18,681 cases of deaths from malignant diseases were notified, including 1,057 cases due to malignant diseases of lymphatic and hematopoetic tissues. Of these 3,362 (18.0%) had been residents of the district of South Württemberg-Hohenzollern. Adjusted for twelve months, this would amount to 55.7 percent or

1,877 cases of the deaths reported, a satisfactory result for the first year. According to preliminary results, the 3,600 line is exceeded for 1972, even though the number of cases residing outside the district of South Württemberg-Hohenzollern is higher than in 1971.

2.2. Distribution by Sex

Whereas the percentage of deaths is 51.2 for the female sex, the registry contains 68 percent. This is due to the high participation rate among gynecologists.

2.3. Nationality

The population includes 8.8 percent of foreigners, and the registry includes 1.5 percent. This is not surprising because there are few foreigners in the age groups in which cancer occurs.

2.4. Age

Registry cases are relatively younger than the cases recorded in mortality statistics. This may be conditioned by the nature of the recording system (hospitals cases only). Older people are probably less intensively examined than younger patients. The high rate of participation among gynecologists also contributes to the divergent age distribution.

2.5. Residence

One of the primary aims of the registry, the determination of the regional distribution and more-than-coincidental accumulation of cancer cases ("clusters"), cannot be achieved. In the course of territorial reforms, so many counties have been subject to geographical alterations and so many towns and villages shifted administratively from one county to another that comparisons with earlier data are no longer possible. In addition the boundaries of the counties have changed as of January 1, 1973, and changes on a community level are being continued. For this reason a more detailed evaluation according to residence must be left to a later date.

2.6. Diagnosis

The diagnoses are coded according to the 8th revision of ICD. Malignomas of the female reproductive organs are substantially more strongly represented than in statistics on causes of death thanks to the high rate of participation of women's hospitals, and also because of the more favorable prognosis.

For example, death statistics list carcinoma of the cervix uteri in only 1.7 percent of all cases, but in the registry, this site, including carcinoma in situ, represents the maximum for a single localization, with 15.9 percent.

2.7. TNM System

Data are available for 83.7 percent of all cases. As shown by inquiries, some of the units participating first started TNM classification under the influence of this registry. Stage T_1 included:24.4 percent of carcinomas of the stomach (n=164), 27 percent of the colon cases (n=51), 22.9 percent of cancers of the rectum (n=109), 49.2 percent of the breast cancers (women only; n=189), 64 percent of cancers of the corpus uteri (n=114), 28 percent of malignomas of the ovaries (n=76). Due to a misunderstanding, the stages for lymph node involvement and distant metastases were not evaluated.

2.8. Types of Malignomas

Carcinomas comprised 87.1 percent, sarcomas 2.9 percent.

2.9. Histological Findings

Evaluation caused considerable difficulties as there is no standardized nomenclature. The data of one type starts out from the cell type (e.g. flattened epithelium) while the other relates to a specific structure (e.g. scirrhus). For the year 1972, coding will be according to the Illustrated Tumor Nomenclature of the UICC. As far as can be anticipated, useful results can be expected. Data on differentiation for 1971 were given with 15.5 percent, for grading with 0.4 percent.

2.10. Reliability of the Diagnosis

The quota of histologically confirmed cases, at 83 percent, is surprisingly high. Undoubtedly this reflects the high rate of participation of operative fields.

2.11. Causes of Diagnosis

Of all cancer cases, 85 percent were diagnosed from symtoms, and only 5.7 percent by screening methods; in 1.2 percent data relating to diagnosis are missing. None of the 109 cases of carcinoma of the rectum or of the 37 cases of cancer of the prostate was detected by screening methods, but this holds true for 1 percent of the 76 cases of malignomas of the ovaries, 2.6 percent of the 114 cases of cancer of the corpus uteri, 7 percent of the 44 cases of lung cancer, 9 percent of the 189 cases of breast cancer, and 33.5 percent of the 197 cases of carcinoma of the cervix, including carcinoma in situ. For 1972, provision is made for a classification according to stages, depending on the cause of diagnosis.

3. Final Remarks

The quality of any registry depends essentially on the degree of participation and the exactness of the data supplied. However, if participation is voluntary, control is inevitably limited. It seems to be very important to inform participants of results as soon as possible. The main benefit of the registry will not really become apparent until it is possible to establish the directions and degrees of trends. But every series must have a starting point and every beginning is far from easy, especially under the given circumstances. A particular objective of the registry is to contribute to the evaluation of cancer screening. As the TNM classification has been broadly accepted, it is possible to compare stages of cancers detected by screening methods with those detected by symptoms, especially for the sites covered by the health insurances' screening program.

Studies of Epidemiology

Contributions of Cancer Registries to Epidemiological Research

J. Clemmesen

Epidemiological results emanating from cancer registries, apart from those of cancer registration in general, vary with the type of neoplasm in question. It may therefore be most practical to subdivide them according to the site of neoplasm.

Rare Neoplastic Diseases

In principle, the detection of rare neoplasms offers the best conditions for full benefit to be derived from cancer registration, but registries have only rarely been established under circumstances offering this possibility. Nevertheless, it was achieved with outstanding success when the Cancer Registry in Kampala, Uganda, established by J. N. P. DAVIES and his associates, reported a frequent occurrence of jaw tumors (8) and were able to furnish data for Burkitt's studies on multicentric jaw tumors, which proved to be a frequent manifestation of the juvenile African lymphosarcoma. Burkitt's mapping out of the geographical distribution of his tumor was therefore facilitated largely through the Kampala registry.

Cattle Leukosis

It may be pertinent in this connection to mention the mapping of cattle leukosis in Denmark, where Bendixen was able to demonstrate the uneven distribution of epizootic leukosis, in contradistinction to juvenile leukosis, both in cattle. Systematic registration has now made a campaign directed at the complete elimination of the disease possible, which is currently in full swing and having considerable success.

Testis

Any rare neoplasm with well-defined characteristics is a good subject for an efficient registration system, but if results with a bearing on epidemiology are to be obtained, it is vital that the detection of the tumor is fairly uncomplicated and also that its incidence is irregular, either in space, as in the case of Burkitt's lymphoma and cattle leukemia, or in time, as in that of carcinoma of the testis. The frequency of this neoplasm has been negligible in most countries. It was observed in 1958 (10) that mortality rates for United States whites show an excess peak about the age of 35 to 40 years over non-whites. In non-whites there is then a gradual increase in frequency, which from 55 years coincides with the rates for whites. The rates given by these authors and cohort studies on English mortality data (5) suggested that the incidence of this neoplasm was rising.

Since figures published by the Danish Cancer Registry showed incidence rates in excess of all other published rates, analysis was carried out.

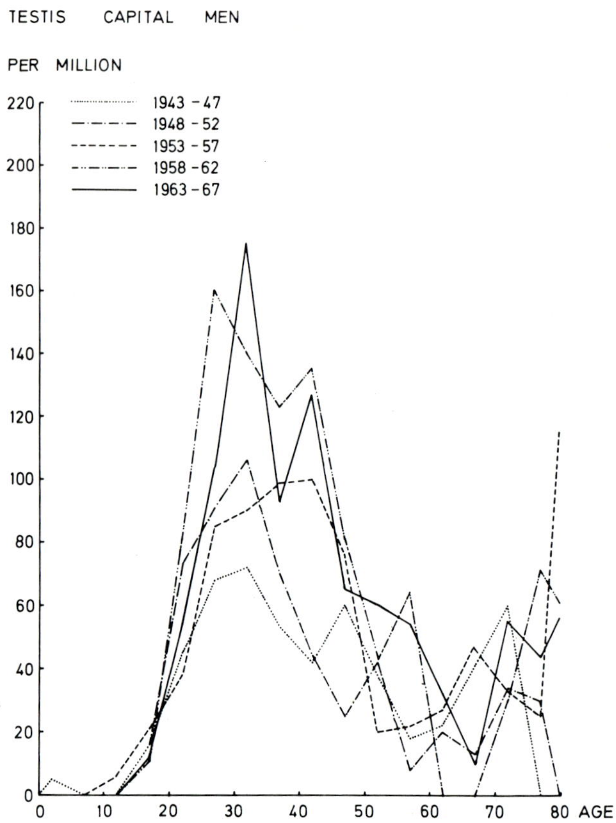

Fig. 1

It appeared that in Denmark, rates had almost doubled during a period of 20 years, particularly those for men in Copenhagen. This increase in cases was limited to the age peak between 20 and 50 years, which also decided the international differences. The Danish rates were the highest on record.

This is as far as registration can bring us at the moment. We have a pretty good idea of the various incidence levels of regions with cancer registration, but until some specific factor can be incriminated, or until some further means of investigation is developed, we cannot hope for progress.

As already mentioned, epidemiological studies based on registration are only possible when a change in incidence is in progress. Theoretically, a decrease in numbers might be expected to present as much opportunity as an increase, but this is probably not the case in practice. After all, the detection of a factor that has been added to the environment is more difficult than the identification of something that has disappeared.

More Frequent Neoplasms

Lung

Carcinoma of the lung used to be a fairly infrequent neoplasm, and an increase in the number of cases was observed as early as 1912. However, there was some controversy as to whether this was a genuine increase or only an apparent one resulting from better diagnosis, the elimination of tuberculosis and the extensive introduction of radiography of the lungs having some part in this.

When the Danish Cancer Registry opened in 1942, one of its tasks was to examine the reality of the increased incidence of lung cancer.

The question was answered by a comparison of mortality rates and incidence rates from the Cancer Registry against rates based on the radiography screening program of the Tuberculosis dispensary.

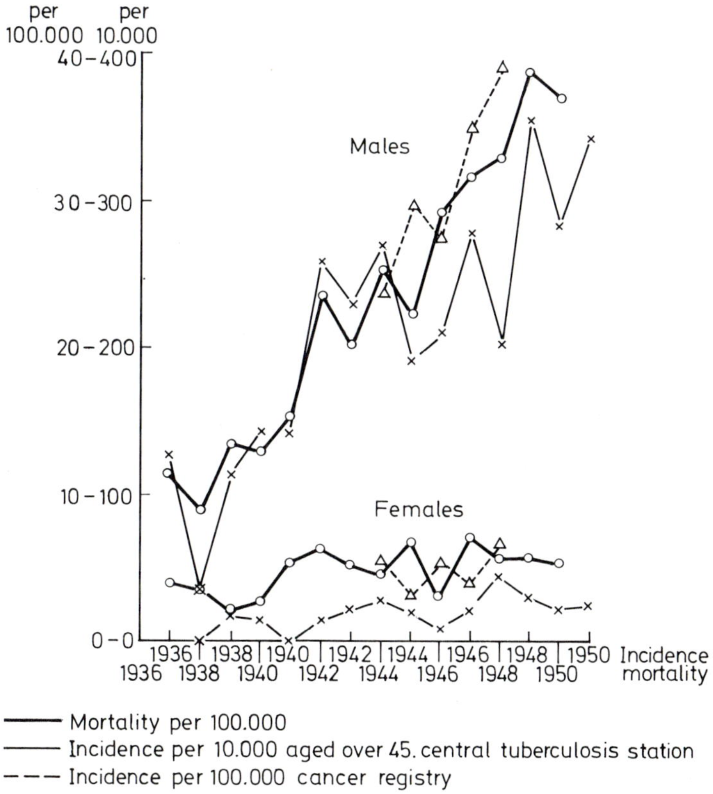

Fig. 2.
Lung cancer in Copenhagen, 1936-1950

The figures show crude mortality rates per 100,000 inhabitants for Copenhagen for the years 1936-1950 (solid line) and the incidence rates of the Cancer Registry (dotted line) for the years 1943-1950. The two curves are quite compatible, considering that diagnosis and notification of the registry will take place rather more than one year before death on average.

Rates based on the data from the Tuberculosis Dispensary have been restricted to persons over 45 years to avoid undue bias resulting from the intensive radiographic screening of e.g. teenagers during the period concerned. In addition, incidence has arbitrarily been given per 10,000 inhabitants.

It is striking that the frequency of bronchial carcinoma diagnosed from radiograms in persons examined for tuberculosis has increased exactly in parallel to the general incidence in the city.

This result is as near an approach as is possible to proof that the increase in cases reported is not due to improvements in diagnostic methods. In support of this conclusion it should be mentioned that the percentages of hospital admissions (about 93), biopsy-confirmed cases (about 67), and postmortem examinations (about 60) remained the same during these years. Another piece of evidence is that even if all deaths that occurred in Copenhagen during 1921 to 1923 among men aged 45-64 years and were ascribed to pneumonia and bronchitis were assumed in fact to be lung cancer, their annual total would not equal the lung cancer death rates observed for 1953.

It may be of interest to note that in the original study the curves did not coincide, and this was interpreted as an argument against the reality of the increase. However, when we checked on the fresh data from the Tuberculosis Station a few years later, we were surprised to find that they did coincide. On inquiry we learned that all radiographs had been revised on the basis of later experience. With a view to the

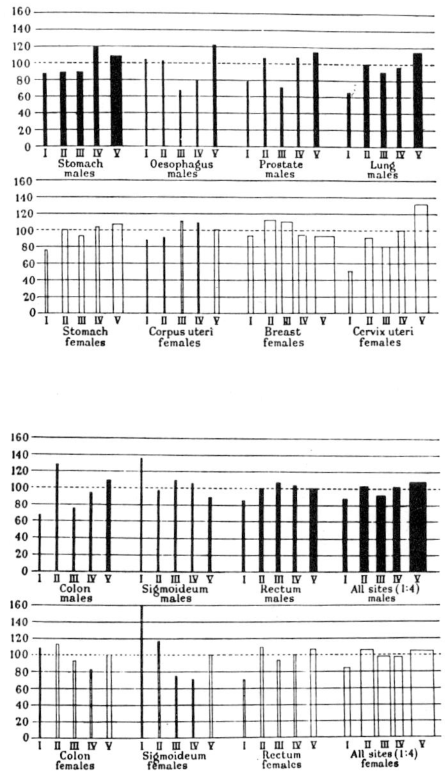

Fig. 3. Standardized incidence for malignant neoplasms of various sites in groups of subdistricts according to annual rental given as percentage of values expected. Copenhagen, 1943-1947

alternative diagnosis of tuberculosis all findings of tubercle bacilli and all postmortems on persons filed with the Tuberculosis Station had been checked.

A further contribution from cancer registration was provided at this stage of lung cancer epidemiology by a study on the social distribution of cancer cases in Copenhagen.

For this study we took advantage of an administrative subdivision of the city into 22 subdistricts for taxation purposes. Various items of information were available for these subdistricts, such as age distribution of the population and the average annual rental. The subdistricts were then grouped into five classes by rental, on the assumption that this was a better indicator of socio-economical standard than income. This would probably no longer be the case because various steps have been taken to counteract the social effects of differences in rental.

The percentage of the average value varied between 66 percent for the wealthiest class through 99, 90, and 97 for the middle classes, to 116 for the poorest quarters of the city. It is true that the findings were based on small numbers, but they were later confirmed by a revision of English data and in an American study. Social factors can be many things, including, as we now know, cigarette smoking. At the time these findings suggested that the decisive factor in the increased incidence of lung cancer was an exogenic one.

The registration data contained more information.

Mortality data from various countries showed that the increase in lung cancer began in the lower age groups, moving to older groups as the years went on and as the younger groups passed into older ones. Thus, a group born in a certain year would show higher rates than the group born the year before and the following ones would gradually show still higher rates. This strongly suggested that the oncogenic factor began its influence with a particular generation, while an overall influence such as air pollution might be expected to raise rates for all age groups at the same time.

This increase by cohorts opened a way for the computation of prognosis. Since the curves for the different cohorts (Jahrgänge) all run parallel, it seems justified to assume that prolongation of the last could allow an opinion on the final values to be reached, provided the development continued as it had started.

Our computations gave the result that when the cohort which then showed the highest rates for men, i.e. men born around 1905, had reached the age of 80, which would happen in 1985, the value for lung cancer incidence in Copenhagen would be roughly the same as that for all malignant neoplasms in 1945. Since this prognosis was worked out in 1953 there has been a slight retardation in the increase, which has probably been counterbalanced to some extent by a rise in the average age of the population.

Thus, while it has been possible for a cancer registry to present some results bearing on the epidemiology of lung cancer, mortality statistics have been able to yield much the same, although not with the same degree of reliability. Cancer registration has, however, made it possible to follow one neoplasm from the time it was a fairly rare disease to the present day, when it has become one of the most frequent neoplasms.

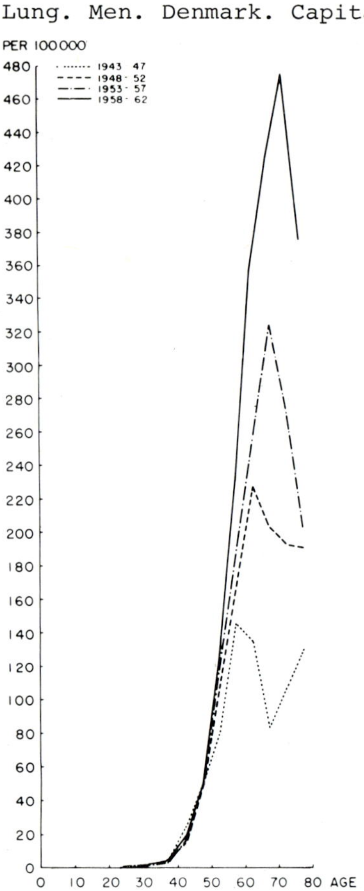

Fig. 4

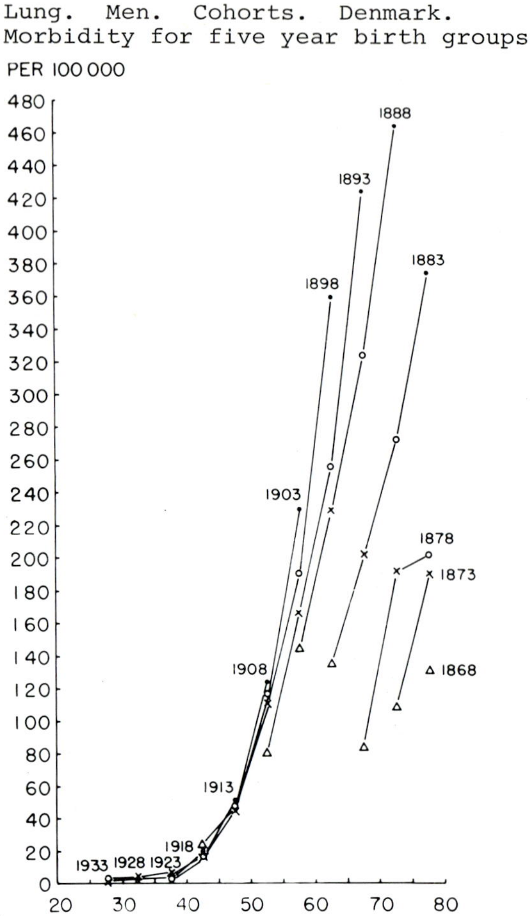

Fig. 5

Fig. 4. Lung cancer morbidity among men in the capital of Denmark. Age distribution for 5-year periods. 1943-1962

Fig. 5. Lung cancer morbidity among men in the capital of Denmark. Morbidity for five-year birth groups. 1943-1962

Computed annual number of deaths	
1951-55	241
1956-60	362
1961-65	507
1966-70	660
1971-75	808
1976-80	919
1981-85	979
1986-90	1,007

Fig. 6. Prognosis for cancer of lung. Copenhagen, 1953

Another neoplasm has, however, been followed with the aid of cancer registries from its first appearance in epidemiology up to the present, namely cancer of the urinary bladder. Although it can be said that the facts would have emerged in the absence of cancer registries, it is also true that they would have been revealed if cancer registries had been the only means of research.

Neoplasms of the Urinary Bladder

In 1955 a review of the data from the Danish Cancer Registry showed, unexpectedly, that rates of incidence for papillomas and carcinomas of the urinary bladder were rising in Copenhagen. Hospital doctors had centralized cases on urological wards, and although they had noticed higher numbers they were inclined to believe that the increase was only apparent.

It should be mentioned at this point that the registry had insisted from its inception that all cases of papilloma should be reported, whether histologically proven to be malignant or not. The fundamental assumption was that if left untreated all papillomas would become malignant, so that statistics planned with a view to epidemiology would have to take them all into account. It would be difficult to prove that all cases ultimately become malignant, since it would be impossible to show that there was no malignancy without removing the entire papilloma.

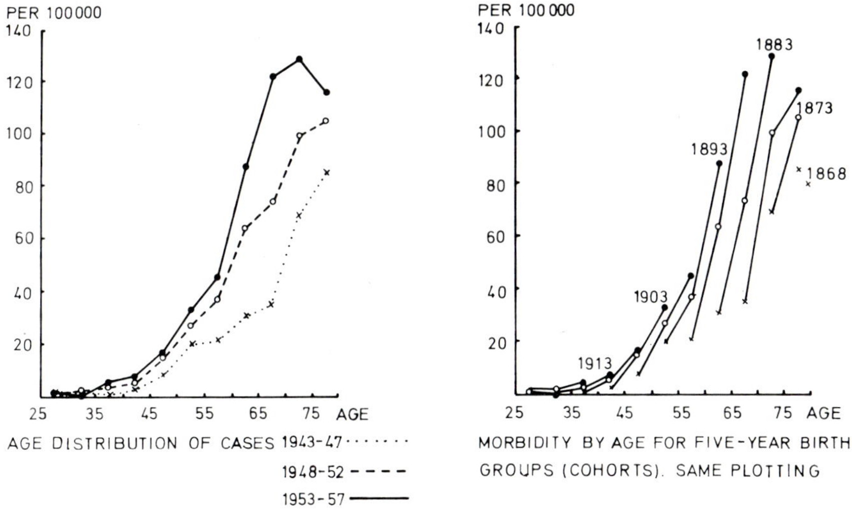

Fig. 7. Urinary tract, men. Copenhagen, 1953

It also appeared that the increase in rates for bladder tumors, like the increase for lung cancer, was most pronounced in Copenhagen, and for men. An apparent increase in men in provincial towns and rural areas at the same time was questionable, and rates for women had been constant, although slightly higher in the capital than elsewhere.

The similarity in pattern to the increase in lung cancer was striking to everybody (3) and an inquiry into the smoking habits of the patients available in Copenhagen from the files of the registry was immediately begun, later resulting in a monograph (15), preceded by a number of preliminary reports.

About the same time, a study based on clinical records and investigating the smoking habits of patients with bladder tumors (14) pointed strongly to the need for confirmation from another source, and special studies on a minor scale (9) and a large-scale prospective study (11) pointed to a correlation between bladder tumors and smoking.

Contemporary cohort studies (5) suggested that the mortality of bladder tumors was increasing, and it may be argued that these studies would also have been carried out without cancer registration. However, it is questionable whether they would have been as convincing, in view of the various sources of error to which mortality statistics are subject and the scepticism voiced at the time against studies into lung cancer and cigarette smoking. No such criticism was levelled against the studies on bladder tumors.

Similar studies have also been carried out in Leeds with reference to both lung cancer and bladder tumors. In England, the excellent studies by Case and his co-workers have shown a considerable incidence, expressed in the mortality, of occupational bladder tumors. Other workers, however, failed to demonstrate any association between bladder tumors and tobacco smoking for men in Leeds (1). Although Doll maintains that the reality of an association with tobacco has now been found in his prospective study of British doctors, the incidence in smokers amounting to about twice that expected in nonsmokers, there may be other aspects to the question as occupational exposure is low in doctors. It was observed on the basis of Danish registration data that the incidence of bladder tumors among men in Copenhagen is rising in a pattern of cohorts, much as the incidence of lung cancer has. It was difficult, however, to take the similarity in the pattern for granted, because bladder tumors tend to affect older age groups than lung cancer does, and since the increases incidence of both makes it impossible to compare the actual age curves the basis for comparison must be the average age curve for the cohorts.

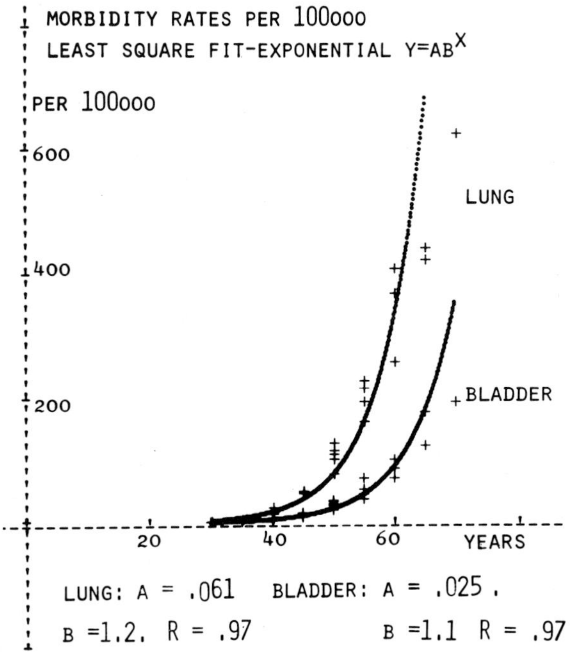

Fig. 8. Lung cancer and urinary bladder neoplasms by age, men born later than 1895. Copenhagen, 1943-1967

The construction of these age curves, which may be termed the true age curves, necessitates access to accurate data for a uniform and settled population over a reasonably long period of some years; these requirements are fulfilled by the material recorded on men in Copenhagen for 1943 to 1967.

Data for this population, calculated for five-year birth cohorts, have been fed into a computer programmed for the calculation of the best approximation of an arbitrary number of observations to the simple exponential function $y=ab^x$ by means of the method of least squares.

With the correlation coefficients found (Spearman's R=0.97 for lung and 0.97 for bladder,) the approximation between the points observed and the hypothetical curve is as close as can reasonably be expected from clinical data.

This similarity in age distribution between the two neoplasms, at least under conditions like Copenhagen's, allows determination of the difference between the two in average age at onset, expressed as the ages at first diagnosis. Calculations show that the age curve for bladder tumors begins and ends 9.3 years later in life than the lung cancer curve, at the age of 47, and 10.5 years later at the age of 64. Since most workers have accepted an average period of induction of about 20 years for lung cancer, the assumption of a corresponding period of 30 years for bladder tumors would quite consistent with our experience so far.

In view of the variation between countries and even cities in the causes of bladder tumors, it may be dangerous to generalize from these results. It is fair to say, however, that up to now occupational tumors of the bladder have not been demonstrated in Copenhagen, although attention has been drawn to the possibility of it.

Conversely, the difficulties in demonstrating any association between bladder tumors and tobacco smoking in England might be assumed to be due to excessive occupational exposure that tends to wipe out the less pronounced effects of tobacco.

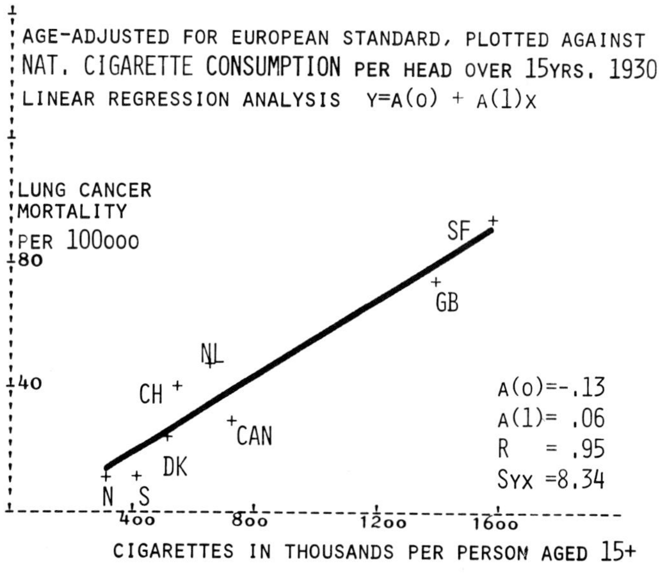

Fig. 9. Lung cancer mortality. Europe and Canada. 1950, per 100,000

Consideration of the time when the increase in lung cancer was largely limited to the male sex reveals that mortality rates were associated with the amount of cigarettes smoked in the country in question about 20 years earlier. Diagram 9 illustrates this correlation on the basis of an adjustment for differences in age distribution in the various countries. Earlier presentations have failed to make this adjustment, so that Great Britain and Finland were placed in the opposite order. It should be added that these countries were the only ones shown in the diagram where an increase had been observed for females.

A corresponding diagram made up from figures recorded ten years later for tumors of the urinary bladder fails, however, to show a corresponding pattern, and the obvious conclusion is that this may be due to differences in occupational exposure. The morbidity rates reported for bladder neoplasms by the nation-based cancer registries in Denmark, Norway, and Sweden are exceptional in that they show a linear progression suggestive of a correlation when plotted against national consumption of cigarettes 30 years earlier. (R=0.99, S=0.54).

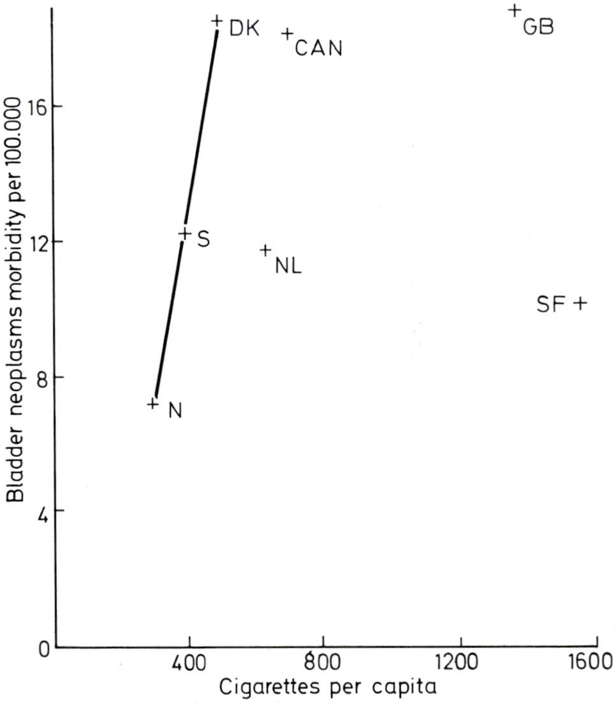

Fig. 10. Bladder neoplasm morbidity in various countries, per 100,000 men, 1960, age-adjusted European standard, against national cigarette consumption per head in 1930

As already mentioned, it is easier to use data from registries for the recognition of the epidemiology of cancers that are increasing in incidence, than for that of established cancers for which we must assume oncogenic exposure affecting large numbers, if not the entire population, for as long as man can recollect. This negative experience applies in particular to cancer of the large intestine, including the rectum, and to a lesser extent to cancers of the stomach. Nonetheless, the demonstration of international differences in incidence, as reported by registries, may yield valuable information. In the case of cervical and endometrial cancer of the uterus, and of mammary cancer, the outlook is more promising, due to their connection with hormonal issues. From its inception, it was possible for the Danish Cancer Registry to contribute data on these cancers for genetic studies undertaken on our initiative in collaboration with the late Professor T. Kemp, of the University Institute of Human Genetics, Copenhagen.

One study on mammary cancer (12) showed an excess of cases among sisters and mothers of patients. It is true that this was not confirmed in England, but there is every reason to assume differences in the genetics of the English and the Danes.

Analysis of the age distribution curve revealed a hook about the age of the climacterium. Further analysis confirmed that while mammary cancer as a whole is more frequent among unmarried than among married women, this applies only to the postclimacteric age groups. Four studies by different authors have reported an excess of married patients before the climacterium, although this is not statistically significant. Nevertheless, I would be inclined to believe in its reality. On this basis it seems quite reasonable that the crossing of the two curves at the climax can differ between countries and regions and from time to time, which may explain the variations in the behavior of the hook.

As a curiosity revealed, or at least finally demonstrated, by registration, it may be mentioned that mammary cancer is slightly more frequent in the left than in the right breast with a ratio of 107 percent. However, relatives of women with a cancer in the right breast show a tendency to right-sided dominance with a ratio of 7 : 2, while the corresponding ratio for left-sided cases is 2 : 8. This difference may be due to a genetically determined asymmetry in the amount of glandular tissue.

Genetic studies on cervical and endometrial cancers of the uterus (4) showed an excess of cases among sisters although not among mothers of patients with cervical cancer. An excess of esophageal carcinoma in their fathers was also observed. All this might be explained by the social grading demonstrated in the aforementioned study on the socioeconomic distribution of cancer in Copenhagen, which is unfavorable to the poor. It is true that similar gradings had previously been found in England on the basis of mortality data, but less efficient treatment among the poor could contribute to higher mortality.

Although the numbers of endometrial cancer cases were too small for statistical significance, they tended to show an excess of cases among sisters and mothers of patients, which is compatible with the clinical observation that these cases often develop in the presence of hormonal abnormalities.

The earliest contribution to epidemiology emanating from a cancer registry was probably a publication that demonstrated the association between cervical cancer and syphilis on the basis of data from Upstate New York (13). A later study from Copenhagen (16) confirmed the suggestion that both diseases were associated with an excessive frequency of sexual intercourse.

The contributions of cancer registries to epidemiology are naturally not restricted to these clearcut examples, but have in many cases been woven into studies extending to other fields, like the comparison of leukemia age curves between Brooklyn and Copenhagen, or the calculation of cervical cancer morbidity among Jewish women. If we extend the epidemiology of cancer as far as that of infectious diseases, we should include the assistance of cancer registries in the organization of mass screening projects, or e.g. the calculation of the improvement in survival rates for mammary cancer brought about by a campaign in Denmark for breast self-examination (Fig. 11).

Breast   Denmark   Women

0 - 44 YEARS

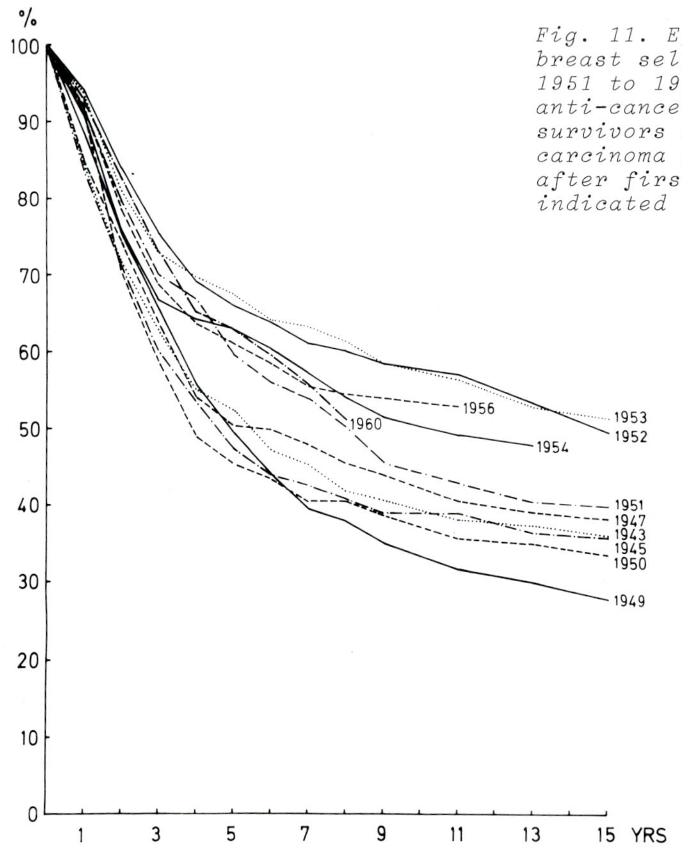

Fig. 11. Effect of a campaign for breast self-examination conducted 1951 to 1954-55 by the Danish anti-cancer league; percent of survivors among Danish women with carcinoma of breast up to 15 years after first attendance in the year indicated

A more negative result was the demonstration on the basis of the data from the Danish registry that a considerable decrease in the numbers of cases of gastric cancer reported from rural areas was only apparent and due to improvements in diagnostic technique.

Some workers would describe the result of applying registry data to the question of clusters of leukemia as equally negative, as it is only too easy to conclude that cancer registration has had the same effect on these as electric light on ghosts. Nevertheless, since most cancer registries have been established in industrialized regions we are inclined to forget that such areas may not offer the same conditions for the transmission of an agent, e.g. a virus, as rural Africa, where a cluster on semicontinental scale has been irrefutably demonstrated.

It is therefore to be hoped that cancer registration will be developed under as widely varying conditions as possible, but also that a blind belief in the benefits of uniformity will not succeed in eliminating different methods of collecting and disseminating information. If we insist too much on international uniformity we could replace enterprising national research with sterile international administration.

References

1. ANTHONY, HONOR, THOMAS, GRETTA: Bladder tumors and smoking. Int. J. Cancer 5, 266 (1970).
2. BENDIXEN, H. J.: Studies of leukosis enzootica bovis. U. S. Publ. Health Service, Publ. No. 1422, 1965.
3. BIERING, G.: Blærekræft - Lungekræft. Ugeskrift for Læger 1409, (1955).
4. BRØBECK, O.: Heredity in Cancer uteri. Aarhus: Universitetsforlaget 1949.
5. CASE, R. A. M.: Cohort analysis of cancer mortality in England and Wales 1911-54 by site and sex. Brit. J. Prev. soc. Med. 10, 59 (1956).
6. CLEMMESEN, J.: Statistical studies in the aetiology of malignant neoplasms. Acta path. microb. scand. Suppl. 174 I,II (1965). ibid. Suppl. 209 III in press Suppl. 247 IV (1969).
7. CLEMMESEN, J., BREMERSKOV, V.: Parallel morbidity age curves for neoplasms of lung and bladder. Biomedicine, 19, 198 (1973).
8. DAVIES, J. N. P., DAVIES,: Tumours of the jaw in African children. Int. Cancer Congress, 1958. Acta U. I. C. C. 16.
9. DENOIX, P. F., SCHWARTZ, D.: Tabac et Cancer de la vessie. Bull. Cancer 43, 387,(1956).
10. GRUMET, R., MACMAHON, B.: Trends in mortality from neoplasms of the testis. Cancer (Phil.) 11, 790, (1958).
11. HAMMOND, C., HORN, D.: Smoking and death rates. J. Amer. med. Ass. 1294-1308, (1958); 1159, (1966).
12. JACOBSEN, O.: Heredity in Breast Cancer. Copenhagen: Nyt Nordisk Forlag 1946.
13. LEVIN, M. L., KRESS, L. C., GOLDSTEIN, H.: Syphilis and cancer. New York State J. Med. 42, 1737 (1942).
14. LILIENFELD, A., LEVIN, M., MOORE, G.: The association of smoking with cancer of the urinary bladder in humans. Amer.med. Ass. Arch. int. Med. 98, 129, (1956).
15. LOCKWOOD, K.: On the etiology of bladder tumours in København-Frederiksberg, Acta path. microb. scand. Suppl. 145 (1961).
16. RØJEL, J.: The interrelation between uterine cancer and syphilis. Acta path. microb. scand. Suppl. 97 (1953).

Pointers from Regional Variation in Incidence – International Perspectives

C. S. Muir

There are several classes of regional variation in cancer incidence, which will be examined in turn with reference to their value for epidemiological cancer studies

International Differences

The cancer incidence map of the world reveals how little information is available - vast areas are still terra incognita. The most useful compendia of data are those which have been collated and presented in a standard format by the International Union Against Cancer (39, 40). The second of these two volumes covers 58 populations in 24 countries throughout the world and includes several African populations, the various migrant groups in Israel and the different ethnic groups resident in South Africa, Alameda County (California), El Paso (Texas), New Zealand, and Hawaii. For mortality the most useful data are those compiled by SEGI et al. (30). Relative frequency material has also been reviewed (43, 8).

Despite the inadequacy of our knowledge, the differences known to exist between cancer levels in many parts of the world have always been intriguing.

Such variations can be used to formulate and test hypotheses, and if they are soundly based, even the crudest of generalizations can lead to conclusions of major importance. Thus, Kennaway, examining primary liver cancer in the Bantu population of southern Africa and in Negroes in the United States, concluded that "the very high incidence of primary cancer of the liver found among negroes in Africa does not appear in negroes in the United States, and is therefore not of a purely racial character. Hence, the prevalence of this form of cancer in Africa may be due to some extrinsic factor, which could be identified" (16). On the other hand, the extreme rarity of testis cancer in negroes, whether resident in the United States, the Caribbean or Africa, is still difficult to explain on environmental grounds (37).

It has been postulated on the basis of geographical differences in cancer incidence (11) that some 80 percent of human cancers are likely to be due to environmental factors and thus, at least theoretically, preventable when the causes are identified. These conclusions are based on comparison of the highest and lowest recorded incidence for a given cancer site, on the assumption that the observed difference was due to environmental agents. Migrant and other studies have shown the majority of such differences are not likely to be due to genetic factors.

Lung cancer exhibits a marked geographical variation in incidence, but virtually all studies show a close link between cigarette smoking and lung cancer no matter where they were conducted (41), which suggests that this habit is universally harmful although to different degrees.

A controlled study in Brazil, Greece, Japan, Taiwan, Wales, the United States, and Yugoslavia (22) revealed that although a pregnancy at an early age conferred some degree of protection against breast cancer, this did not account for all the observed international variation in risk, indicating that other factors must be involved. The further finding that, contrary to entrenched belief, lactation history has no influence on breast cancer risk is all the more impressive for being demonstrated in seven countries (23).

Any theory of etiology must, if complete, be in consonance with observed geographical variation. Cancer of the prostate is rare in Japan, being seven times more common in Canada. Thus the supposition expressed in a Canadian report (34), that sexuality, and in particular extra marital activity, are linked to the neoplasm seems an inadequate explanation for the wide differences observed.

Thus, in summary, inter-country variation in incidence should lead to etiological hypotheses and may provide a means of testing these. In addition, any theory of causation that cannot explain the observed geographical differences must be incomplete or wrong.

Correlation Studies

Studies correlating cancer incidence in several countries and a variety of environmental factors in the same countries are becoming increasingly popular. Cancer of the prostate has been found to be correlated with tea and coffee consumption (35), bone cancer with alcohol consumption (29), cancer of the esophagus with alcohol consumption (38), and so on.

Such results are notoriously difficult to evaluate; the consumption of tea and coffee are linked to many other aspects of the environment, any one or combination of which may be the "true" causal agent. Chance associations are to be expected and the values obtained in the correlations can alter considerably with different registries. Thus the close correlation obtained between nasopharyngeal cancer and population density disappears if Singapore, a country which has very high values for both, is excluded from the set of countries considered. Many of the environmental variables available, such as meat consumption *per capita*, are of a questionable precision, and furthermore are *usually not* available at the individual level.

Intra-Country Differences

It is not always easy to compare data coming from different countries. Age-adjustment cannot standardize for differences in methods of data collection, medical customs and differences in language and training.

Chap. II of Vol. 2 of Cancer Incidence in Five Continents (40) indicates how widely cancer registries differ in their practices and procedures. While such biasing factors could be expected to be less pronounced within a country than between countries, there has been a tendency to ignore regional differences in cancer levels within a country.

The incidence of thyroid cancer for 1963-1966 is significantly higher for Scotland than for the rest of Great Britain (12). Multiple myeloma is reported to be twice as common in northeast Scotland as in the remainder of Scotland and England and Wales. Lip cancer (ICD 140) is commoner in males in Scotland and southwest England than in the rest of Great Britain, but in females this cancer is much commoner in southeast England. It has been suggested that variation in lip cancer reflects different occupational exposure in males and sunbathing in females.

While such regional differences, like international ones, would usually need to be confirmed, their existence is nevertheless most important to an international Agency and other workers, in that they may be very useful in the testing of specific hypotheses. Thus a sharp gradient in esophageal cancer frequency on the shores of Lake Victoria between West Kenya and neighboring parts of Tanzania and elsewhere was noted (5). To test the hypothesis that the differences were due to congeners in home-brewed beers, COLLIS et al. (4) examined alcoholic drinks from these regions for the presence of nitrosamines; none were found, suggesting that some other factor is involved.

For an examination of the relationship between aflatoxin consumption and human liver cancer, LINSELL and PEERS (14) chose an area in Kenya (the Murang'a district) which, with a considerable range of altitude, possessed climatic characteristics favoring the growth of *Aspergillus flavus* to varying degrees. The dietary intake of aflatoxin was measured by cooked meal sampling and the incidence of liver cancer was recorded. The preliminary results show considerable parallelism. Although similar results have been reported from Thailand (31) these studies do not by themselves prove aflatoxin to be a human carcinogen.Areas with high aflatoxin intake and no liver cancer, and vice versa, should be sought, bearing in mind the possible role of hepatitis virus (27).

Intra-country differences are likely to be smaller in developed countries. Few regions of the world can offer contrasts such as those observed in the Caspian Littoral of Iran (18), where within a distance of 500 km the annual age-adjusted incidence rate for esophageal cancer varies from 110 to 17 in males and from 170 to 6 in females.

Geographical studies within a country can be undertaken at levels other than the total population. One study (21) used the records of the medical department of the railway systems of India, a country where there are eight zonal railways running a group of 86 railway hospitals for railway staff throughout the subcontinent. Gastric cancer was found to be common in the South and rare in the North, whereas primary cancer of the liver was common in the North, an inverse association considered to indicate an unspecified dietary etiology. There must be many other such opportunities.

In some countries, specific regions are largely inhabited by discrete tribal groups. Tribal differences have been observed in the incidence of malignant melanoma of the foot in Ugandans (20). Examinations of the soles of feet of persons attending hospitals throughout the country showed that the tribal frequency of discrete small black areas of pigment with clearcut margins paralleled that of malignant melanoma. This example illustrates the use of a geographical difference to confirm a suspected association.

Urban-Rural Differences

Urban-rural comparisons are a special type of intra-country study. Thus, in 1964-1966 the age-adjusted incidence rates for lung cancer for males in urban areas in Norway (25.2*) were much higher than those

---

*age-adjusted rates per 100,000 per annum - adjusted to the world population distribution (UICC, 1970).

for males in rural districts (10.5*). Similar but smaller differences were seen in females (4.2* and 2.2* respectively) (26). In several countries such variations have often been ascribed to atmospheric pollution, but they could well be due to other environmental factors, such as differences between town and country dwellers in smoking habits, asbestos exposure, etc. Nevertheless the existence of such risk differentials does permit testing of the atmospheric pollution hypothesis.

With urban drift, urban-rural differences are tending to become less distinct in many countries. The towns contain many persons who have spent part of their life in the country, a circumstance which may condition subsequent disease risk (9, 28).

Not all urban-rural differences lead to a testable hypothesis. A two-fold difference in the incidence of testis cancer between males resident in Copenhagen and in the rural areas of Denmark (3) is as yet unexplained.

It is also necessary to consider intra-country differences in an international manner. It might make more sense to consider river basins, plateaux, coastal regions, and mountain zones rather than department, province or country. While computer techniques that permit complex analyses and recombinations do exist (13, 1), unfortunately the cancer registration data that are suitable for such processing are often not available.

Cancer of the colon and rectum are considerably more common in Denmark than in Sweden (15), but when it is realized that the part of Sweden close to Denmark has higher rates than the rest of the country (in contrast to gastric cancer) the problem becomes much more interesting and complex.

Thus, although environmental differences are likely to be less striking, systematic demonstration and exploration of intra-country differences are considered necessary as the problems of standardization and logistics are likely to be smaller than those at the inter-country level.

It may be asked why variation within a country is of international importance rather than being of purely local concern. The answer is that a solution to one's own cancer problems may be much more easily found in another country. Groundnut products are consumed in substantial quantities in much of Europe and North America. Such products contain varying amounts of aflatoxin, which may be a human carcinogen. Is it better to wait and see whether primary liver cancer increases in the importing countries or to determine the risk in a population known to have a high primary liver cancer incidence and to eat aflatoxin-contaminated foodstuffs? The benefit is not all one way. Many developing countries are industrializing and changing their dietary patterns. They can benefit by research on the associated cancer risks conducted elsewhere.

Migrants

International migration is of primary importance in that the study of migrants permits assessment of the effect of movement from one environment to another, and indirectly the extent of the involvement of racial and genetic factors (9). While for a few migration involves minimal environmental change, the migrations which have taken place in the past century have generally involved considerable changes in diet, way of life, etc. A list of the migrant populations currently available for study has been published (32), KMET has analyzed the cancer risks in migrant groups and suspected factors arising from such studies in tabular form (17). In view of the potential gain from migrant studies it is very regrettable that for various reasons many countries do not wish to keep accurate records with the place of birth and duration of stay in the host country.

When cancer registration exists in both the host country and the country of origin, the potential of migrant studies is considerably expanded.

As most migratory movements have been towards areas with better medical and statistical facilities, the cancer data on migrants may be much better than those for the population in the country of origin. However, migrants are rarely a representative sample of any population.

Intra-country migration is commonplace. The existence of such groups originating from different regions of Colombia in Cali, a city with a cancer registry, has been used to show a correlation between stomach cancer incidence and the prevalence of gastric-intestinal metaplasia (6).

Variation within Sites of Malignancy

Comparison of cancer risk is usually based on the rubrics of the International Classification of Diseases published by WHO (43). While these rubrics generally deal with one organ taken as a whole, provision has been made for anatomical divisions within organs such as skin, stomach and colon (ICD 153), but only a few countries, e.g. Canada (33), and certain cancer registries publish to this degree of detail.

While malignant melanomas of skin (ICD 172) are distinguished from other malignant neoplasms of skin (ICD 173) and choriocarcinomas have their own rubric (ICD 181), the one internationally accepted cancer classification has not yet made provision for the coding of morphology.

Although examination of the distribution by anatomical subsite or histological subtype may not seem to have much value in the formulation of etiological hypotheses from a purely local point of view, when taken in conjunction with international differences they may not only suggest causal hypotheses but be used to test them.

Thus, analysis of the anatomical distribution of skin cancer has disclosed European, Asian and African patterns (25, 2). The high proportion of lower-leg skin cancer in Africa has been attributed to tropical ulcer, burns, etc., whereas the European pattern of head and neck skin cancer, with a high proportion of basal cell carcinoma, is related to the genetically determined lack of melanin protection against ultraviolet light.

Over 90 percent of cancer of the bladder in Natal Africans is squamous, whereas the proportions in Natal Indians, in Birmingham (UK) and in Sweden are 50 percent, 13 percent, and 2 percent respectively (36). Taken individually, these frequencies have comparatively little meaning; together such wide divergence points to the likelihood that there are different etiological exposures in these regions, schistosomiasis being widely suspected as the cause of the squamous cancers so common in much of Africa. The differences between Birmingham and Sweden might be artefactual, but examination of the characteristics of persons with squamous cancer in these registration areas could be rewarding.

It is well known that gastric cancer exhibits considerable geographical variation. The disease is now known to have two significant histological variants, the diffuse and the intestinal (19). The hitherto rather disappointing case-control dietary studies for gastric cancer might be much more rewarding if repeated for these two types of the disease, as it could be that the effect of the causal factor for one of the variants would be diluted out when aggregating what may be in effect two different diseases.

Rare Cancers

Some problems may be only soluble at the international level. This is particularly true for industrial exposure. It is said that 20,000 new chemical substances enter the environment each year and there is rarely any warning to the public in general that they are now exposed. The persons most at risk are likely to be those manufacturing the chemicals in question, so that careful detailed records of employment and processes on which employed are essential for workers in the chemical industry. Modern technology is such that the number of persons so exposed in any one country, let alone in any one plant, may be relatively low. The need for international collation of registries of exposed persons thus becomes even more pressing.

Comment

Variation is the life-blood of the cancer epidemiologist. The difficulties there would be in studying the etiology of lung cancer in a world where everybody smoked 10 cigarettes a day are evident.

The more widespread cancer registration becomes, the more likely regional variations are to be discovered, in that the nature of the environment is determined in no small measure by geographical position. The basis of geographical epidemiology is the existence of reliable incidence data (7), but very little is available. Obviously a reliable cancer registry is not built in a day and registries deserve the long-term support not only of the epidemiologists but also of other members of the oncological world. But cancer registries must never allow themselves to become hoarders of data or custodians of graveyards of dead statistics. By participating in local and international studies they can ensure that their data are properly used and their unique value recognized.

Before demanding and encouraging the creation of new registries we should be sure that existing risk differentials are being fully exploited. As stated elsewhere (24), the descriptive epidemiologists, which includes those looking at regional variation from an international standpoint, have been slow to realize that the demonstration of a geographical difference in cancer can no longer by itself be regarded as sufficient. The reasons must be examined, and quickly, in conjunction with scientists in other disciplines.

It might be thought that a disease such as cancer which has an "incubation period" of up to twenty years would permit a leisurely pace of progress. This is not so. The environment can change very rapidly, even in the most primitive parts of the world. It is possible that many current studies measuring events and linking them to present cancer levels are already too late.

Acknowledgements

I wish to thank my colleagues for helpful criticism and Mlle A. Broc for typing the manuscript.

References

1. BURBANK, F.: Patterns in Cancer Mortality in the United States: 1950-1967. National Cancer Institute Monograph No.33. Washington D.C.: Govt. Printing Office 1971.
2. CAMAIN, P., TUYNS, A. J., SARRAT, H., QUENUM, C., FAYE, I.: Cutaneous Cancer in Dakar. J. Nat. Cancer Inst. 48, 33 (1972).
3. CLEMMESEN, J.: Statistical studies in the aetiology of malignant neoplasms. Acta path. microbiol. scand. Suppl. 174, Vol. III (1969).
4. COLLIS, C. H., COOK, P. J., FOREMAN, J K., PALFREYMAN, J. K.: Cancer of the oesophagus and alcoholic drinks in East Africa. Lancet 1972 1, 441.
5. COOK, P.J., BURKITT, D. P.: Cancer in Africa. Brit. med. Bull. 27, 14 (1971).
6. CORREA, P., CUELLO, C., DUQUE, E.: Carcinoma and intestinal metaplasia of the stomach in Colombia migrants. J. Nat. Cancer Inst. 44, 297 (1970).
7. DOLL, R.: Prevention of Cancer. Pointers from Epidemiology. The Rock-Carling Lecture, p.30. London: Nuffield Provincial Hospitals Trust 1967.
8. DUNHAM, L. J., BAILAR, J. C.: World maps of cancer mortality rates and frequency ratios. J. Nat. Cancer Inst. 41, 155 (1968).
9. HAENSZEL, W., KURIHARA, M.: Mortality from cancer and other diseases among Japanese in the United States. J. Nat. Cancer Inst. 40, 43 (1968).
10. HAENSZEL, W.M., LOVELAND, D.B., SIRKEN, M.G.: Lung cancer mortality as related to residence and smoking histories. J. Nat. Cancer Inst. 28, 947 (1962).
11. HIGGINSON, J.: Present Trends in Cancer Epidemiology. In: Proc. 8th Canadian Cancer Conference, Honey Harbor, Ontario. p. 40, 1968.
12. HILL, G. B., HOWITT, L. F., SOAPER, A.: Cancer Incidence in Great Britain 1963-1966. Office of Population Censuses and Surveys, (Studies on Medical and Population Subjects No.24). London: H. M. S. O. 1972.
13. HOPPS, H. C., CUFFEY, R. J., MORENOFF, J., RICHMOND, W.L., SIDLEY, J. D. H.: The computerized mapping of disease and environmental data. Mapping of Disease Project 1968.
14. IARC: Annual report 1970, p. 87. Lyon; 1971.
15. DE JONG, U. W., DAY, N. E., MUIR, C. S., BARCLAY, T. H. F., BRAS, G., FOSTER, F. H., JUSSAWALLA, D. J., KURIHARA, M., LINDEN, G., MARTINEZ, I., PAYNE, P. M., PEDERSEN, E., RINGERTZ, N., SHANMUGARATNAM, K.: The distribution of cancer within the large bowel. Int. J. Cancer 10, 463 (1972).
16. KENNAWAY, E. L.: Cancer of the liver in the negro in Africa and America. Cancer Res. 4, 571 (1944).
17. KMET, J.: The role of migrant populations in studies of selected cancer sites: a review. J. chron. Dis. 23, 305 (1970).
18. KMET, J., MAHBOUBI, E.: Esopahgeal cancer in the Caspian Littoral of Iran: initial studies. Science 175, 846 (1972).
19. LAURÉN, P.: The two histological main types of gastric carcinoma: diffuse and so-called intestinal type carcinoma. Acta path. microbiol. scand. 64, 31 (1965).
20. LEWIS, M. G.: Malignant melanoma in Uganda. Brit. J. Cancer. 21, 483 (1967).

21. MALHOTRA, S. L.: Geographical distribution of gastro-intestinal cancers in India with special reference to causation. Gut 8, 361 (1967).
22. MCMAHON, B., COLE, P., LIN, T. M., LOWE, C. R., MIRRA, A. P., RAVNIHAR, B., SALBER, E., TRICHOPOULOS, D., VALAROAS, V. G., YUASA, S.: Age at first birth and breast cancer risk. Bull. WHO 43, 209 (1970 a).
23. MCMAHON, B., COLE, P., LIN, T. M., LOWE, C. R., MIRRA, A. P., RAVNIHAR, B., SALBER, E., TRICHOPOULOS, D., VALAROAS, V. G., YUASA, S.: Lactation and cancer of the breast. Bull. WHO 42, 185 (1970 b).
24. MUIR, C. S.: Geographical Differences in Cancer Patterns. In: Doll, R., Vodopiji, I., Eds. Host-Environment Interactions in the Aetiology of Cancer in Man - Implementation in Research. Scientific Publication No. 7. Lyon: IARC (In press).
25. National Cancer Institute: Conference on Biology of Cutaneous Cancer. NCI Monography No.10. Washington: US Govt. Print. Office 1963.
26. PEDERSEN, E.: Cancer Incidence in Norway. In: UICC (1970) loc. cit., p. 238.
27. PRINCE, A. M., LEBLANC, L., KROHN, K., MASAYEFF, R., ALPERT, M. E.: Detection of SH antigens in sera of patients with chronic active hepatitis, cirrhosis and carcinoma of the liver. Lancet 1970 2, 717 (1970).
28. REID, D. D.: Bronchitis among the British. Israel J. med. Sci. 7, 1569 (1971).
29. SCHWARTZ, D., LASERRE, O., FLAMANT, R., LELLOUCH, J.: Alcool et cancer. Etude de pathologie géographique portant sur 19 pays. Europ. J. Cancer 2, 367 (1966).
30. SEGI, M., KURIHARA, M., MATSUYAMA, T.: Cancer mortality for selected sites in 24 countries, No. 5 (1964-1965). Sendai: Tohoku University School of Medicine 1969 (gives data for a further 17 countries).
31. SHANK, R. C., BHAMARAPRAVATI, N., GORDON, J. E., WOGAN, G. N.: Dietary aflatoxins and human liver cancer. IV. Incidence of primary liver cancer in two municipal populations of Thailand. Fd. Cosmet. Toxicol. 10, 171 (1972).
32. STASZEWSKI, J., SLOMSKA, J., MUIR, C. S., JAIN, D. K.: Sources of demographic data on migrant groups for epidemiological studies of chronic disease. J. chron. Dis. 23, 351 (1970).
33. Statistics Canada: New primary sites of malignant neoplasms in Canada (as reported by Provincial Tumour Registries). Catalogue 82-207. Ottawa: Information Canada 1972.
34. STEELE, R., LEES, R. E. M., KRAUS, A. S., RAO, C.: Sexual factors in epidemiology of cancer of the prostate. J. chron. Dis. 24, 29 (1971).
35. STOCKS, P.: Cancer mortality in relation to national consumption of cigarettes, solid fuel, tea and coffee. Brit. J. Cancer 24, 215 (1970).
36. TULINIUS, H.: Frequency of some morphological types of neoplasms of five sites. In: Cancer Incidence in Five Continents. loc. cit., p. 23, (1970).
37. TULINIUS, H., DAY, N. E., MUIR, C. S.: The rarity of testis cancer in negroes. Lancet. 1973 1, 35.
38. TUYNS, A. J.: Cancer of the oesophagus; further evidence of the relation to drinking habits in France. Int. J. Cancer 5, 152 (1970).
39. UICC: Cancer Incidence in Five Continents. Vol. I. Eds DOLL, R., PAYNE, P., WATERHOUSE, J. Berlin-Heidelberg-New York: Springer 1966.
40. UICC: Cancer Incidence in Five Continents. Vol. II. Eds DOLL, R., MUIR, C., WATERHOUSE, J.: Berlin-Heidelberg-New York: Springer 1970.

41. US Public Health Service: Smoking and Health. Report of the Advisory Committee to the Surgeon General of the Public Health Service. Washington, D.C.: US Govt. Print. Office 1964.
42. US Public Health Service: The Health Consequences of Smoking. A Report to Surgeon General. Washington, D.C.: US Govt. Print. Office 1972.
43. WHO: Manual of the International Statistical Classification of Diseases, Injuries and Causes of Death. Vol. I. 8th Revision. Geneva: WHO 1967.

The Comparability of Cancer Incidence Rates

G. Linden

Background

The California Tumor Registry was organized in 1947 to obtain data on the occurence of cancer in the California population and to provide information on the extent of disease, treatment and survival of cancer patients. Hospital participation is entirely voluntary but the number of hospitals participating has had to be restricted because of financial limitations. Thirty-four of the 48 hospitals presently participating in the Registry have been in the system for more than 25 years. The Registry now has 400,000 cases on its records, with 20,000 new cases being added each year. These constitute about one third of the estimated 60,000 new cancer cases in California each year.

Although the hospitals participating in the Registry are generally representative of all hospitals in California, the cancer cases reported from these hospitals cannot be related to any defined population. A population-based registry was therefore established in one county, Alameda County, and cancer incidence data have now been compiled for this population of 1,000,000, starting with cases first diagnosed in 1960.

The National Cancer Institute of the United States has conducted three cancer surveys in ten metropolitan areas of the United States, in 1937, 1947, and 1969-1971. The San Francisco Bay Area in California is one of these ten areas, and the 1969-1971 survey was carried out under the direction of the California Tumor Registry. The five counties encompassed in this area had a population of 3,000,000 in the 1970 census, including about 360,000 persons of Spanish-American background, 330,000 blacks, 88,000 Chinese, 44,000 Filipinos, 33,000 Japanese and 12,000 American Indians. Data on cancer incidence will soon be available for the years 1969, 1970 and 1971.

A continuing Cancer Incidence System in these same five counties has been organized, starting with cases first diagnosed in 1972. This operation is being carried out under the Tumor Registry and Cancer Incidence Section of the newly organized San Francisco Bay Area Resource for Cancer Epidemiology.

We have made one basic change in the organization of the incidence system. Cancer registries are generally unable to obtain current incidence rates, partly due to delays in obtaining information on extent of disease and treatment. As a result, most cancer incidence rates are not available until one to two years after the close of the data year. The need for current cancer incidence rates is increasing because of the introduction of many new factors into the environmental system without precise knowledge of the possible carcinogenic effects. The use of food additives, new food processing methods, increased use of hormones, radiation, and chemicals and the increasing pollution of air, water, and the general environment make it imperative to develop data systems that will allow prompt detection of changes in cancer incidence. We have therefore instituted a Rapid Reporting Cancer Incidence System. Data are obtained from each hospital at the time of patient discharge, and contain only the essential information needed, i.e. demographic data, date of first diagnosis, primary site, and histologic type. The goal of the system is to produce preliminary incidence rates three months after the end of a calendar year and final rates six months after the end of the year. Organization of this system was started in May - June, 1972. Despite the late start, by April 1973 we had obtained 98 percent of the 1972 cancer cases estimated for the 75 hospitals in the five-county area. Computer matching of deaths from cancer against the incidence file has been carried out and preliminary incidence rates have also been computed. Further case finding and querying of cases took place over the next few months, and final cancer incidence rates for the year 1972 were available by July 1973.

Comparability of Cancer Incidence Rates

There is general agreement that cancer incidence rates are needed to assess the magnitude of the cancer problem and to provide basic information for describing variations in cancer incidence among various population groups and geographic areas. Such data can and have already provided valuable clues to the possible cause or causes of cancer. The data must, however, be valid and comparable from one geographic area to another and from one time period to another if they are to be useful. Data that are not comaprable (and we cannot always be aware of this) will generate false clues that waste time and energy and distract from the valid and important clues.

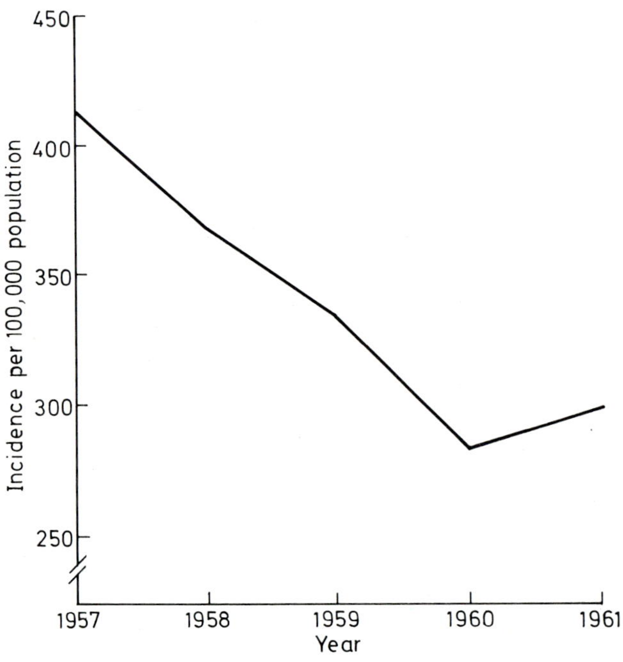

Fig. 1. Age-adjusted cancer incidence rates per 100,000 population all sites, 1957-1961

As an example, Fig. 1 shows the trend in cancer incidence rates in a speciific geographic area. These are actual data taken from a publication (the dates have been changed). The graph shows that the cancer incidence rate for all cancer was more than 400 per 100,000 population in 1957 and then decreased to less than 300 per 100,000 population by 1961. Truly remarkable this represents a 25 percent decrease in cancer incidence in four years. If the data were valid and we knew what had caused the decrease, it would be a time for great rejoicing. Unfortunately, there is a less happy explanation, which will be discussed later. It is especially disconcerting that the authors made no comment and gave no explanation for the apparent sharp decrease in total cancer incidence rates.

The problems of comparability of cancer incidence rates are not new; they have already been described and discussed. The editors of the first volume of "Cancer Incidence in Five Continents" (1) have discussed some of the problems, and this discussion was expanded in Volume II (2). An excellent article based on a specific registry is also available (3).

Cancer Incidence Rate

A cancer incidence rate can be defined as the rate at which new cancer cases arise in a specified population during a given time period. The numerator of the rate shows the number of new cancer cases, while the denominator shows the population at risk. The rate is usually given per 100,000 population for a given year.

The equation is simple enough, but the elements in it are difficult to define and determine. Cancer is easily definable in general terms, but difficult when reference must be made to specific inclusions and exclusions. There are several coding schemes in existence, each with its own basic rules, definitions of malignant and benign tumors etc.

It is also necessary to define what is meant by a "new" cancer case. The most desirable definition would be a case at the point when the first cell changes occur, but we have no way of determining this point in the development of the disease and probably could not obtain agreement on the exact point at which the change took place. Date of onset of the disease is another point at which new cases could be counted, but this phrase is open to many interpretations and difficult to apply in a mass data system. Date of diagnosis, date of treatment, date of hospital or clinic admission, date of pathologic verification, date of discharge, date of death, date of recording of the case are other possible points of reference (2).

The bottom half of the equation shows the population at risk. Population data are generally obtained by census at regular or irregular intervals in various countries. The validity of these data can be questioned; it is difficult to be sure whether all persons are counted. Various problems are encountered in the definition and enumeration of racial, ethnic, religious and other subgroups in the population. Estimation of the population for intercensal years is equally complex. Many countries and smaller geographic entities contain populations which migrate frequently from one area to another. Valid estimates of such populations by age, race, social class, etc. five, seven or nine years after a decennial census are hard to achieve.

Completeness of Reporting

It is generally agreed that incidence rates should be based on a complete count of all cases. Completeness of reporting is very difficult to achieve even under the best of circumstances (and in most areas of the world the best of circumstances do not exist). Cancer patients may not be hospitalized, their diagnoses may not be accurate, the disease may not be diagnosed until the time of death and then not properly recorded on the death certificate.

If it is hard to achieve completeness of reporting, it is equally difficult to evaluate it, since there are no definitive standards against which the completeness of reporting can be measured. This is an area that needs further exploration.

Prevalence Versus Incidence

We have described incidence as the rate at which new cases occur in a given population. Since it is not possible to determine the exact time at which a malignancy begins, we are forced to use the time when the disease is diagnosed. This time of diagnosis is influenced by medical, emotional and social factors, and may differ to a considerable extent from one patient to another since the time between the beginning of a malignancy and the diagnosis is generally lengthy and varies considerably by primary site and histological type.

Prevalence of cancer refers to the cancer cases existing in a population at a given point in time, regardless of when they were diagnosed. Unfortunately, it is not always easy to differentiate prevalence cases from incidence cases, and prevalence cases are often included in the calculation of incidence rates. This mixture provides an explanation of the data shown in Fig. 1. Previously diagnosed, recurrent hospital cases, plus all those who died of or with cancer but were not admitted to a hospital during the period of Registry operation were included in the "incidence" rates shown in the graph. It is obvious that the previous diagnosed hospital cases should not have been included, but one suspects that the inclusion of these non-hospital cancer deaths also contributed to the artificially inflated rates during the first years. Care must be taken, especially during the first few years of an incidence system, to exclude deaths for patients initially diagnosed prior to the first year of the data system. Failure to do so increases the number of prevalence cases counted as incidence as surely as the inclusion of previously diagnosed hospital cases. The number of previously diagnosed (old) cases and cancer deaths diagnosed prior to the beginning of the system will diminish as the current file of new cases develops.

Cancer cases which represent the prevalence of the disease may intrude in more subtle ways into the computation of cancer incidence rates. A change in the method and time of diagnosis and in the frequency of use of a new technique may cause prevalence cases to be counted as if they were incidence cases. Fig. 2 shows this in a simplified way.

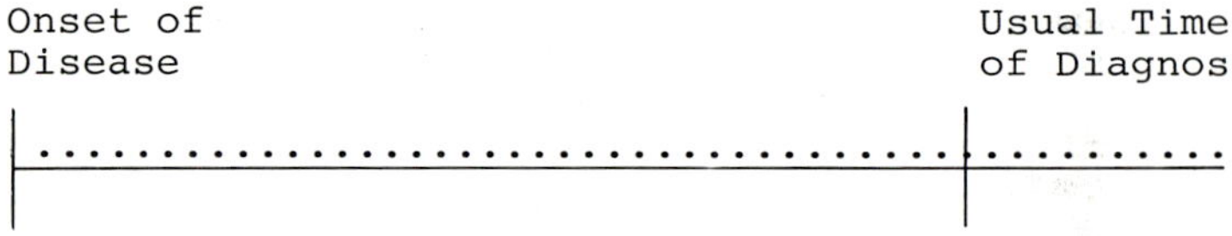

Fig. 2

At any given time, the population will contain persons at different points in the development of the disease. Generally, each person will be diagnosed when his disease becomes clinically evident and will be counted from that time as a case (with considerable variation in time, depending on the site and type of malignancy, level of medical practice, etc.). The diagnosis of cancer at an earlier point in the disease process (this may be a matter of years) will pick up cases that would not ordinarily have been diagnosed and counted until a much later time. These are prevalence cases, not incidence.

Cytology for cervical cancer is designed to find cancer while it is still in the in-situ phase. (Two thirds of cervical cancers being reported to the California Tumor Registry are in situ.) The process, however, will also pick up preclinical invasive cases. Even if the cases with carcinoma in situ are excluded from the calculation of cancer incidence rates (as they should be), the preclinical invasive cases, which are really prevalence cases, will artificially increase the incidence rates. On the other hand, if even a fraction of the in-situ cases would have become invasive if left alone, the removal of the carcinoma while in situ would cause a decrease in the incidence of invasive disease in future years. Incidence rates for cervical cancer are therefore almost impossible to interpret now, because of the increasing use of cytology in various populations. Earlier detection of breast cancer and other cancers will have similar effects on incidence rates.

The mixture of prevalence cases with incidence cases can also be caused by changes in surgical practice. For example, an increase (if it occurred) in transurethral resection for prostatic hypertrophy would probably lead to more frequent observations of prostatic cancer. These cases would be counted at an earlier point than usual and represent prevalence rather than incidence cases. The same holds true relative to the amount of tissue removed at surgery; the chance of a malignancy being discovered rises with increasing extent of surgery. More intense microscopic study of surgical specimens will also discover more malignancies than less detailed examination techniques.

Variation in pathologic diagnosis can have a great effect on resulting incidence rates. For instance, pathologists differ among themselves in their diagnosis of a thyroid lesion from an adenomatous goiter to a true adenoma to a carcinoma.

The finding of occult malignancies as a result of autopsy will also influence cancer incidence rates. The proportion of deaths which are autopsied and the extent of both gross and microscopic examination will have a direct bearing on the number of cancer cases "first diagnosed at autopsy" (cases with no suspicion of tumor prior to death).

It is well known that a sizeable proportion of older males have occult prostatic cancer. These are generally slow-growing tumors which might never become clinical. If death occurs (from any cause) and an autopsy is performed, prostatic cancer may be found. As a result, a relatively large proportion of prostatic cancer cases are "first discovered at autopsy."

In discussing whether to include or exclude cases "first diagnosed at autopsy" a few years ago, we decided that they should not be included in incidence rates since they were prevalence rather than incidence cases. Before implementing this decision, however, we decided to contact a number of other registries to determine their views and practices since we were interested in comparing rates. We wrote to about a dozen registries around the world and received widely differing responses. Some felt that the cases should not be included, others felt that exclusion of these cases would artifially reduce the incidence rates, and others felt that it was so difficult to obtain completeness of reporting that these cases should certainly be included. We decided to make no changes in our own system until some resolution of this problem was achieved.

The responses seemed to indicate that the level of medical care in each area was an important factor in determining preference for inclusion or exclusion of these cases. In countries where cancer patients were more likely to be diagnosed and be admitted to hospitals, the group diagnosed only at autopsy was small and relatively unimportant and could be excluded. In countries where the level of medical care was such that a smaller proportion of cancer patients was being diagnosed and admitted to hospitals before death, it was felt that exclusion of this group would negatively bias the incidence rate.

Proposals for Action

The problems of comparability are difficult and will never be adequately solved to everyone's satisfaction, but there are steps that can be taken to increase the validity and comparability of cancer incidence data.

Data from about 50 registries were included in Volume II of Cancer Incidence in Five Continents (2); a number of others are now operative in various sections of the world. The editors obtained a good deal of information about each of the registries that contributed data.

The Editorial Board for Volume III are presently obtaining information from each of the contributing registries. Perhaps the scope could be expanded to encompass additional information describing each registry's practices, inclusions, exclusions, completeness of reporting, population estimation, limitations of the data, and other pertinent information which would enable the researcher to make more valid comparisons. This might be published as part of Volume III.

I should also like to see the establishment of guidelines for computation and publication of cancer incidence rates. This is a suitable task for the International Agency for Research on Cancer and the International Association of Cancer Registries. The I. A. R. C. and the I. A. C. R. should encourage those who produce cancer incidence data and those who use such data to document publications as completely as possible and to take special care not to avoid or ignore obvious or possible biases. This may be more difficult in a short journal article than in a larger publication but it should be done as far as possible.

Realization of these proposals will not be easy and will take many years of close cooperation and collaboration. The members of the U. S. National Cancer Institute's End Results Group spent many years in discussions and workshops before it was possible to produce a well-documented coding system for reporting cancer end results (4), including detailed definitions, discussions of problems, and basic rules for making decisions. Their realization is absolutely necessary, however, if valid, comparable cancer incidence rates are to be produced for use in assessment of the size of the cancer problem and in the epidemiologic exploration of cancer in various populations.

References

1. UICC: Cancer Incidence in Five Continents, Vol. I. Eds. DOLL, R., PAYNE, P., WATERHOUSE, J. Berlin-Heidelberg-New York: Springer 1966.
2. UICC: Cancer Incidence in Five Continents, Vol. II. Eds. DOLL, R., MUIR, C., WATERHOUSE, J. Berlin-Heidelberg-New York: Springer 1970.
3. TEMPLETON, A. C., BIANCHI, A.: Int. J. Cancer 10, (1972). (Bias in an African Cancer Registry.)
4. End Results Section, National Cancer Institute: Code Manual of the End Results Group. 1967.

The Use of Cancer Registry Data in the Investigation of Industrial Carcinogenic Hazards

J. A. Waterhouse

The kind of cancer registry data to be discussed in the context of this title must first be defined. The cancer registry itself is a "population-based" registry, i.e. it possesses a certain definable population or catchment area from which it draws the cases of cancer it registers. Usually the population itself is defined by geographical, or in some cases political or cultural, boundaries, so that often the registry can be referred to as a territorially based registry. Within its confines it should aim to register every case of malignant disease that is diagnosed, and if it is to be of real epidemiological value it should achieve this aim to the extent of well over 90 percent, and preferably over 95 percent.

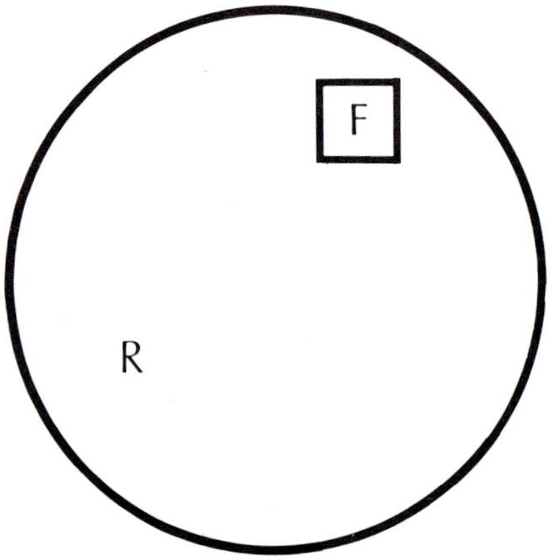

Fig. 1

For convenience, the territorial base of the registry can be represented in a diagram as a circle (Fig. 1), and the registry itself by the letter "R," which can be situated anywhere inside (usually) or outside the territory. The small square labeled F represents the location of a factory within the territory. In the detection of possible carcinogenic hazards at the factory it is necessary to determine how many cases of malignant disease have occurred within a given period of time among people who have been employed there for at least a certain minimum duration of service. The cases of malignant disease found may include those at all sites (preferably) or may be limited to particular sites considered to be of especial importance, and they must be compared with the number of cases that might have been expected to occur on certain simple assumptions, usually that the factory population does not differ in essentials from that of the territory as a whole. If the number of cases of cancer at the factory significantly exceeds the number to be expected it is taken that the basic assumption is in error, and thus that there is an a priori argument for an increased risk in the factory environment.

There are many variations on this fundamental theme of comparison of the observed with the expected number of cases. The method best suited to any particular situation depends on many factors, but primarily on the special circumstances and characteristics of the situation and the degree of sophistication with which they may be matched in the calculation of expectations.

The Registry in Birmingham is a population-based registry drawing its cases from five counties in the West Midlands of England. The map (Fig. 2) shows the division of England and Wales into 15 regions for the purposes of National Health Service administration, and also shows the situation of the Birmingham region and its five counties in relation to the remainder of the country. The population of the region is just over 5,000,000, approximately one-tenth that of the whole country. For the last ten years the efficiency of registration has been of the order of 97 to 98 percent; it is difficult, if not impossible, to be much more precise.

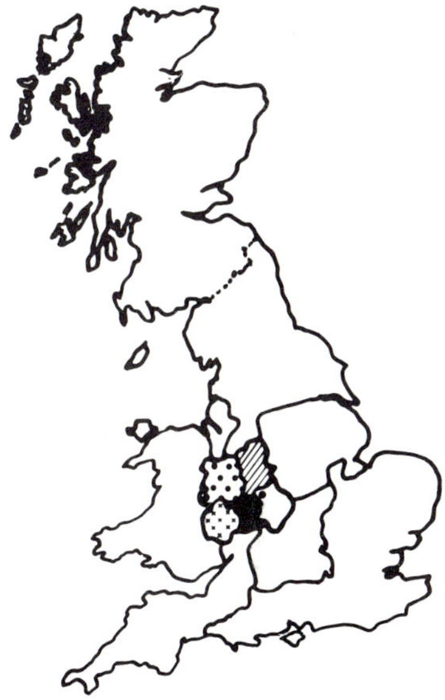

Fig. 2

There is a concentration of industry around Birmingham and in what is known as the "Black Country", mainly to its north. The Black Country got its name from its coal, iron and steel works, many of which persist to this day. In addition to heavy engineering works there are many factories engaged in lighter engineering, in making components for the motor car industry, or indeed in manufacturing cars, especially in the Birmingham and Coventry areas.

Some time ago a discussion with the Medical Inspector of Factories for the Birmingham area led to a review of the numbers of cases we had recorded of epithelioma of the scrotum. This, of course, is well-known for its claim to be the first cancer shown, two centuries ago, to have an occupational origin, when Percival Pott, of St. Bartholomew's Hospital in London, pointed out its high frequency among chimney-sweeps. About a century later it was shown to be associated with shale oil, and then with cotton mule spinning, an occupation centred, for Britain, mainly in the Lancashire area to the north-west of the Birmingham region. A good deal of work was devoted to the study of mule spinners' cancer, and perhaps the best known publication is the monograph by SIDNEY HENRY, first published in 1946, on Cancer of the Scrotum in Relation to Occupation. By that time, however, mule spinning had practically ceased to exist as an occupation, having been superseded by more sophisticated techniques.

There was no mule-spinning in the Birmingham region, but redundant workers from the north may have sought jobs in the region. The graph (Fig. 3) shows the numbers of cases of scrotal cancer registered in the Birmingham registry over a period of about 30 years, and there is a very clear upward trend. With the help of the Registrar General, the number of deaths over a similar period was graphed for the whole country (England and Wales), with a population approximately ten times that of the Birmingham region. The trend for the whole country (Fig. 4) is just as clearly the reverse of ours, and despite the tenfold difference in population size, the national number of deaths and the regional number of cases diagnosed were about the same towards the end of the period. This appeared to justify proceeding further with the investigation.

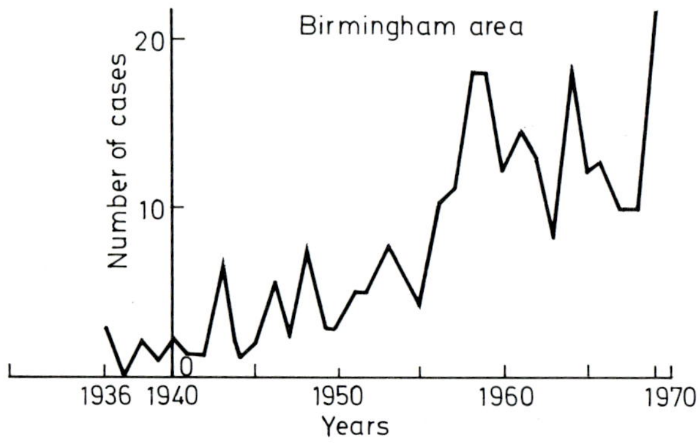

Fig. 3. Epithelioma of scrotum

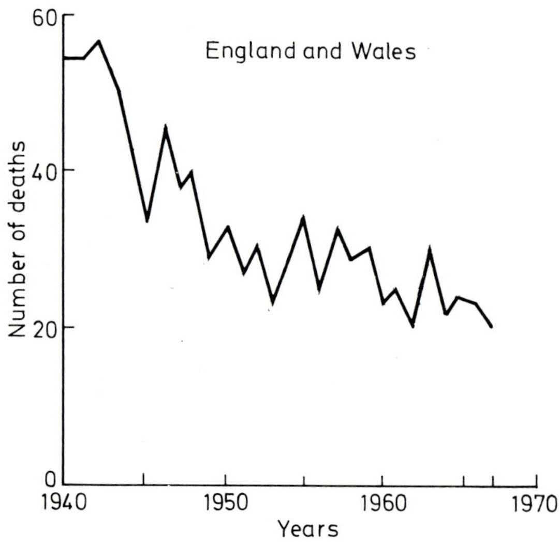

Fig. 4. Epithelioma of scrotum

The cases of malignant disease registered for two other sites of the male genital system, testis and penis, were counted and the totals of cases at all sites obtained; the corresponding figures recorded in the South Metropolitan Cancer Registry were then obtained. This Registry is similarly organized to the Birmingham one, and covers the southern areas of the city of London as well as much of the south and east of England.

Table 1

	BRCR	SMCR	
Population (millions)	4.76	8.22	1.7
Male only	2.35	3.88	1.7
Total cases of malignant disease (3-yrs)	40,069	77,393	1.9
Male only	20,625	38,697	1.9
Total cases of:			
Testis (3-yrs)	152	292	1.9
Penis (3-yrs)	77	139	1.8
Scrotum (8-yrs)	113	55	1/2.1

BRCR = Birmingham Regional Cancer Registry
SMCR = South Metropolitan Cancer Registry

Table 1 compares the figures from the two sources, first for the overall populations, then for cases of malignancy, and finally for the three selected sites. The population figures, being taken from the 1961 Census were a little old, but the 1971 figures were not available. The ratios of numbers between the two registries were nearly two to one, except for the scrotum cases, which were approximately two to one in the reverse direction. This comparison shows, then, that we had about four times the number of scrotal cancers in relation to other sites observed in the South Metropolitan region.

Patients' occupations - which we frequently had to pursue in detail because of deficient information, or changes of job - were then examined, and we found a large proportion of the men worked in the light engineering industry, making such things as components for motor cars and using machines known as "bar automatics". These machines operate largely on their own, performing the several separate tasks involved in the construction of e.g. a hexagonal nut from a long bar of hexagon cross-section by using different tools mounted on a rotatable head. The nut would be bored out, threaded, chamfered, sawn off, and smoothed by successive operations. Apart from feeding the machines with the appropriate bars of metal, the main task involved is the sharpening and re-setting of the tools on the head. This work is done by a small and highly-skilled elite group of workmen known as "tool-setters", who in the course of their work may need to sit astride an oily machine and use oily rags which they keep in their trouser pockets. This small class of tool-setters was the one found to have the highest incidence of scrotal cancers.

I have dwelt at some length on this example, partly for reasons of its intrinsic interest, especially as applying to a site of cancer which has been linked to an occupational cause - or indeed a succession of occupational causes probably for the longest time of any, yet has an extremely low (some people say zero) sporadic frequency of occurrence, but primarily because it constitutes a useful instance of a moderately simple application of cancer registry data in an industrial epidemiological study. Only the numbers of cases classified by site and year were required, first to show the existence of a secular trend, and then to form the basis of a comparison by means of a method of relative incidence. Commonly the use of relative incidence would compare the numbers of cases of one site with those of another for the same period of years, but in this example, while the testis and penis cases were aggregated for a three-year period, the scrotal cases were collected from a period of eight years because of their greater rarity. Since the same periods applied to the various figures from both registries, the overall comparison was not invalidated. Nor were any methods of age-adjustment necessary in the form of comparison that was used, where the contrast was clearcut and obvious.

A different approach to the evaluation of an industrial hazard is exemplified by a study we made of the records of a small factory in the Birmingham region making a certain type of alkaline electric batteries. They had been made at this same factory for a long time but nowhere else. From the meticulous personnel records we were able to note the date each worker was first employed at the factory, his age at that time, and the date when he left - to move elsewhere, or to retire - or died, or whether he was still working there at an arbitrarily chosen closing date to the survey. Only those who had worked for a continuous period of at least one year were included in the survey. We obtained the cause of death for each employee who had died, and searched our register for every one of the total of nearly 250 men who had worked at the factory at any time to discover in which of them cancer had been diagnosed.

By making use of the annual incidence rates of the Registry, classified by site and age, it was possible to compute the numbers of cases of cancer which would be expected to occur in such a group of men followed from their age at entry into the factory until either the date of their death or the closing date of the survey. Thus we were able to compare the numbers of deaths or cases of cancer known to have occurred with the numbers that would be expected if the men were at the same risk as men in the whole of the region.

The hazard to which the men were exposed was cadmium oxide dust. At a recent inquest on a cadmium pigment worker it had been stated that carcinoma of the lung could not be ruled out as a consequence of exposure to dust of cadmium salts. Our actual comparison of observed and expected numbers of cases is shown in Table 2. The overall total expected is much the same as the total observed, and equally there is no evidence for an excessive risk of lung cancer. There is, however, a wide difference between expected and observed numbers of cases for prostatic cancers, and it is statistically very significant. This was an unexpected finding which should be investigated further. This method has the virtue of providing control figures, either from the all-sites total, or from comparisons for other sites not related to the specific hazard under review. It also admits of refinement of application in a number of ways. For instance, the actual period of exposure could be substituted for the time from first employment by deducting from the latter the time spent in other jobs (no longer exposed to the hazard) or in retirement. This of course lowers the ex-

Table 2. Cadmium oxide dust

	Expected	Observed	Probability
All sites	13.13	12	0.660
Bronchus	4.40	5	0.449
Bladder	0.51	1	0.398
Prostate	0.58	4	0.003
Testis	0.11	0	0.898

pected numbers, thus widening the gap between the number expected and an observed excess. In the interests therefore of using a method which minimizes any possible bias in one's favor, and also because there is evidence that even a short exposure may be sufficient to initiate a tumor, it is probably better to use the overall time from first exposure. In the case of rapidly changing incidence rates a cohort method should be applied, and furthermore, where there is wide geographical or social variation in the incidence rates within a region, those appropriate to the circumstances of the actual industry should of course be used in calculating expectations.

A rather different use of cancer registry data in the investigation of industrial carcinogenic hazards is illustrated by an extended examination we made of the scrotal cancer data. One result of the study had been to incriminate mineral oil or one of its constituents as the likely carcinogen, in the form of the cutting oil or a lubricant. A good deal of this oil escaped into the atmosphere to form a mist, which was apparent as a blue haze when one looked any distance down a factory workshop. The question as to whether such oil mist constituted a malignancy hazard, or indeed any kind of hazard, to those working in it had been raised but had remained unresolved for many years. Principally this was because of the inadequacy of the data available for analysis; for cancers, with a time lag of the order of twenty years between exposure and evidence of disease, adequate data would require a quality of records and follow-up that it would be quite unrealistic to expect when men move freely from job to job, and the conditions of exposure show wide variation. A further important consideration is that the likely tumor sites are also commonly found in the general population and it is thus almost impossible to attribute them to the hazard in question with any degree of certainty.

Our patients with scrotal cancers can, however, be regarded as a group, the majority of whom are known to have worked in the kind of factory environment which includes an oil hazard, demonstrated by their development of a scrotal tumor. It is very likely that their exposure to oil mist has also been high. We have therefore taken these men as propositi, or index cases, in terms of their exposure, and examined them to see whether they have developed other primary tumors elsewhere. Table 3 shows our results.

The morbidity rates classified by site and age were used to calculate expected numbers, the ages and periods of follow-up being known for each man from the time of diagnosis of his scrotal tumor, either to the time of his death or to a closing date for the survey. In addition to providing the morbidity data for the computation of expectations, the Cancer Registry, by keeping in regular contact with all former patients through its follow-up section, simplifies the tracing

Table 3. Epithelioma of scrotum

Men with subsequent malignancies	Expected	Observed	Probability
All sites	11.60	32	<.001
Respiratory tract	3.62	11	<.001
Digestive tract	3.56	9	<.01
Skin	1.10	10	<.001
Remainder	3.27	2	

of these men independently of the factory, from which they may have retired many years before.

Examination of the results shows first that the number of cases of cancer is greatly in excess of the number to be expected, and that the sources of that excess are three groups of sites. The sites most likely to be affected by oil mist - by inhalation, by ingestion, and by direct contact - are those in these three groups.

It is not my primary concern, however, to discuss the implications of these findings, but rather the role played by Cancer Registry data in obtaining them. The demands of that role can be summarized on the basis of these three examples. In the case of the first study, the requirements were for a reasonably high registration efficiency, but primarily for <u>unbiased</u> registrations, as between various subdivisions of the male genital system. Differential registration, i.e. different likelihoods of registration for different sites of tumor, is often difficult to detect. The best remedy, which may not be simple, is to increase the overall efficiency of registration of cancer at all sites. The second example required a high efficiency of registration in relation to a known population to allow the calculation of reliable morbidity rates by site, sex and age. In the case of the last example, the requirements now include, in addition to those already mentioned, a long period of collection of data and a good follow-up system. All these features should be characteristic of a good cancer registry, but even if follow-up is excluded a cancer registry can make a valuable, and often a unique, contribution to industrial epidemiology.

The Cancer Registry of Cali Colombia* — Epidemiologic Studies of Gastric Cancer

P. Correa, O. Bolaños, F. T. García, G. Gordillo, E. Duque and C. Cuello

Cancer registration in developing countries offers special research opportunities and presents special problems. Findings in these registries not only provide information about the local situation but may also help in the study of trends observed in other countries. Cancer incidence in wealthy western communities tends to show similarities, and often contrasts with patterns common in developing communities. As an example, high rates for colonic and pulmonary cancer and declining rates for gastric and cervical cancer are as characteristic of wealthy communities as they are uncharacteristic of developing communities. These are good reasons for the encouragement of cancer registration in developing countries. We started our work in Colombia as a cancer survey, which was planned to last approximately 3 years. After the planned survey was accomplished, it became clear that its continuation would be highly beneficial and also quite simple because the personnel had already been trained and their experience could be used to great advantage. This explains why our registry uses a combination of the registry and survey techniques: we gather data for all periods of time, but most intensely during the summer months, when we employ medical students for a survey-type activity. This has proved particularly useful in our set-up; it makes work more interesting and attracts students to the field of cancer epidemiology.

Our registry is directed at the study of incidence as a tool for the study of etiology. The work of the registry is closely related to other work oriented towards etiologic studies, with the emphasis on pathology, clinical findings and field surveys of several types. This paper describes the general operation of the registry and illustrates it by describing some of the work done in the area of gastrointestinal tumors.

Cancer epidemiology studies in Latin America are scarce and generally limited to relative frequency comparisons of hospital series. There are, however, conditions in many Latin-American communities that allow adequate investigations in this field. The population of most cities is well known, and adequate medical facilities provide diagnostic evidence for this type of study. It is usually the organization needed for data collecting and processing that is not available. Our studies have been restricted to circumscribed geographic areas with a well-known population composition and adequate medical facilities. This restriction is necessary due to the size of the country, the poor medical facilities in rural areas, and the lack of adequate descriptive data on the composition of the rural population.

Methods of Cancer Registration

The data reported here were obtained from the city of Cali, located in the Cauca Valley 1000 meters above sea level. The valley is separated from the Pacific Ocean by the western range of the Andes system

*Work supported by Public Health Service research contract PH-43-66-907 from the National Cancer Institute.

and a tropical rainy forest. The latitude of the city is 3° 27' N. The average temperature is 24° C. The city is bounded by the river on the east, the mountains on the west, and by well-demarcated north and south borders set by the municipality in official maps. The valley surrounding the city contains mainly sugar cane plantations and cattle farms.

Most of the adult population of Cali have come from other sections of Colombia, mainly from rural areas skirting the Andes mountains. They represent the centuries-old mixture of Spanish immigrants with small, independent, and ethnologically different Indian communities. Spanish culture is predominant in every sense, and includes the adherence of most of the population to Roman Catholicism. There is also a sizable group of Negroes, originally brought from Africa to Colombia to work in mines and plantations, who after their liberation approximately 150 years ago migrated to the coast and warm valleys. More recently, small groups have migrated from Lebanon, Italy, Germany, and Japan, and Jews have also come from different parts of Europe. Information on the proportionate representation of each racial group in Cali is not available.

A national census carried out on July 15, 1964, enumerated 638,211 inhabitants in Cali. The previous census, conducted on May 9, 1951, showed 241,357 inhabitants in Cali. Until the information recorded in the 1972 census is available there will be no good population data suitable for the calculation of rates. The rates for the first 5 years of registration were calculated by interpolation of data from the last two censuses and were close enough to the last census to be considered accurate. Since 1963, population estimates have been made on a sample basis and are not considered accurate. For these reasons, trends are not considered at present.

The aim of this study is to register all the cases of cancer first diagnosed as such by physicians among residents of the city of Cali. Patients born in Cali, or who had migrated to Cali with the intention of living and working there, were considered residents. Patients coming to Cali for other reasons, including prolonged medical treatment, were considered nonresidents. The records of all medical institutions, pathology departments, clinical pathology laboratories, and X-ray services are reviewed by medical students during June, July and August each year. Simultaneously, medical students personally contact all the physicians known to have a private practice in Cali, review their records, and abstract the necessary information. In addition, death certificates for cases not diagnosed before death are abstracted from the Vital Statistics Office.

Medical students chosen for this part of the survey were trained by the staff of the medical school in the techniques of interviewing and data collecting. Their work was reviewed daily by a statistician assigned to the project. All reports were reviewed for completeness, adequacy, and accuracy of diagnostic information and resolution of conflicting data.

Our studies on gastrointestinal tumors began with the registry findings and they led to other special clinical, pathologic and field studies which will be mentioned in the presentation of results.

Studies on Cancer of the Stomach

Our figures for the first 5 years of registration (1962-1966) showed that the incidence rate of gastric cancer in Cali males was 57.5 per

100,000, second only to Japan (1). We decided to analyze these figures more closely, following the general epidemiologic strategy of narrowing down the field of observation in search of the high-risk group. We did this by examining the rates for the natives and different groups of immigrants to the city and also by subdividing the cases into several histologic types after review of the corresponding slides.

For the calculation of rates specific to each immigrant group, information on the place of birth was used. The population of Cali classified by birthplace according to the national census of July 15, 1964 is given in Table 1, grouped by sociocultural regions. Sociologists from the University of Florida and University of Valle drew up the sociocultural regions (2). These regions are based on natural geographical barriers and historically and geographically determined population isolates (Fig. 1).

Table 1. Population of Cali by birthplace, July 15, 1964

Birthplace	Population
Cali	277,050
Neighboring towns (Valle)	101,418
Antioquia, Caldas	95,442
Cauca	42,539
Upper Magdalena	33,941
Cundinamarca, Boyacá	23.035
Pacific coast	19,753
Nariño	16,706
Atlantic coast	3,782
Other areas of Colombia	16,821
Foreign	7,442
Total	637,929

Obvious differences in population structure were found in the different migrant groups probably reflecting characteristics of the population of origin; immigrants from Cauca, Nariño, and the Upper Magdalena are mainly rural agricultural workers from poverty-stricken areas, while immigrants from Antioquia and Cundinamarca have high proportions of city dwellers (Fig. 2).

For histologic studies the classification of Jarvi and Lauren was used, which distinguishes the following main histologic types: Intestinal, Diffuse, Mixed and Others (3-4).

The histologic material available was reviewed and classified by the system of Jarvi and Lauren. The numerators for age-specific incidence rates were the cancer cases diagnosed during a 5-year period (1962-66); the denominators were taken from the 1964 national census. Because of the differences in age and sex structure of migrant groups, rates were adjusted for age and sex by use of the indirect method, with total Cali rates as a standard. Standardized incidence ratios (SIR) were calculated, with the rates in natives of Cali applied to the population of each migrant group (Cali natives = 100).

Table 2 summarizes our findings. The immigrants from the rural high-altitude south have an excess of all histologic types, most marked for the intestinal type. The immigrants from the coast have lower rates for all types, and especially for the intestinal type.

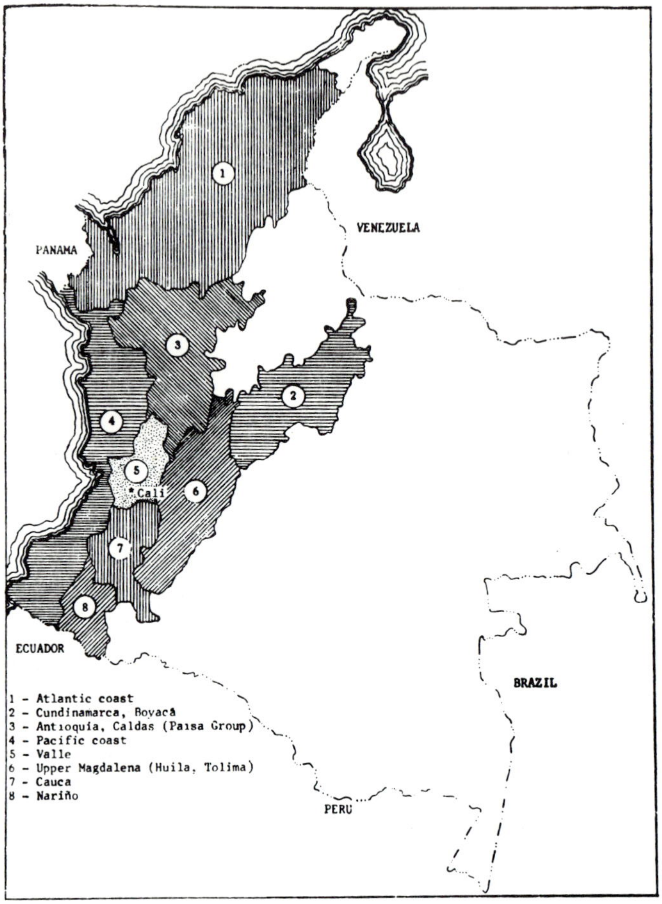

Fig. 1. Map of Colombia, showing the sociocultural areas which represent the main source of migration to Cali. (2)

To link cancer incidence data with the prevalence of lesions that could be precursors of cancer, systematic collection of specimens was begun in Cali in 1966. Approximately 30% of adults dying in Cali are autopsied, mainly in the University Hospital and by the medicolegal service. This report is based on specimens collected from persons dying of all violent causes and most natural causes from the two main hospitals from 1966-68.

Gastric specimens were opened on the greater curvature, attached flat to a board, and fixed in buffered 10% formalin. After fixation, they were examined carefully and thoroughly illuminated with a magnifying lens. Sections were taken from predetermined areas in all specimens. All sections were stained with hematoxylin and eosin and periodic acid-Schiff.

Special attention was given to intestinal metaplasia of the gastric mucosa in view of its possible role as a premalignant lesion. Diagnostic criteria were atrophic mucosa and replacement of normal gastric glands by straight crypts lined with intestinal-type cells. These were

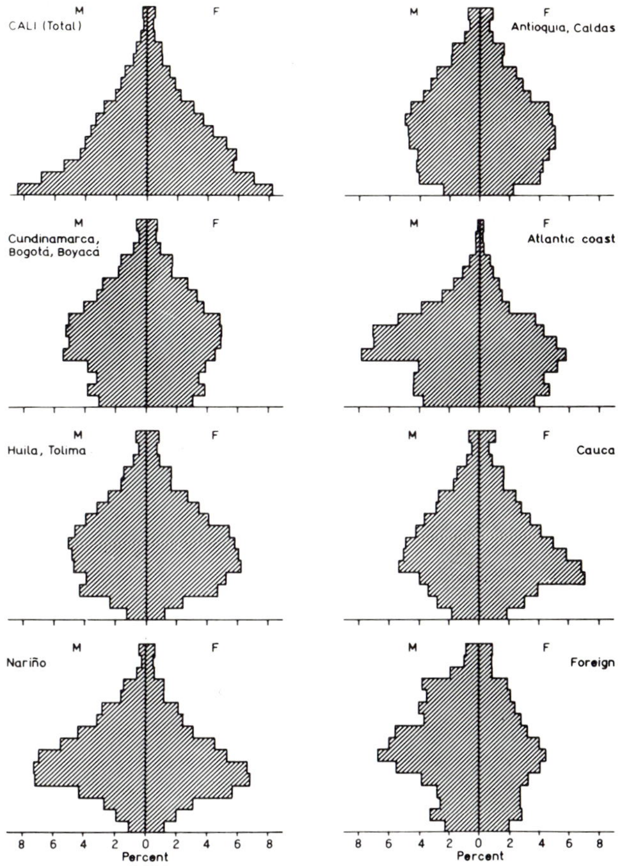

Fig. 2. Population pyramids of the population of Cali (upper left) and its subgroups of immigrants. Each step in the axis of the ordinates corresponds to a 5-year age-group

mainly goblet cells and columnar cells with a striated border. Argentaffine and Paneth cells were also seen occasionally in metaplastic areas.

Lesions of intestinal metaplasia stood out microscopically because they resisted autolysis, whereas the normal glands were autolyzed faster and more severely. Prevalence figures for each migrant group are given in Table 3, which presents crude rates for males aged 15 years and older. A clear gradient was observed, with maximum levels in Nariño, Cauca, and Upper Magdalena that were highly significant in males and in the total population ($P < 0.001$). The number of specimens obtained from migrants from coastal areas was too small for detailed analysis. Hence, a special sample was collected in the coastal city of Cartagena and compared with the other groups. A low prevalence of metaplasia was clearly observed in Cartagena.

These data based on immigrants to Cali, lead us to the conclusion that in Colombia there are areas which represent the extremes of gastric cancer risk. The rural mountaneous area has very high rates, while the

Table 2. Standardized Incidence Ratio (SIR) with 95% Confidence Limits (CL) for Gastric Carcinoma. Total Intestinal and Diffuse Histologic Types by Sex and Birthplace. Residents of Cali, 1962-1966

Birthplace												
Histologic Type	Nariño		Upper Magdalena		Cauca		Antioquia, Caldas		Cali (natives)		Atlantic and Pacific coasts	
	SIR	CL	SIR	CL	SIR	CL	SIR	CL	SIR	CL	SIR	CL
All types												
Both sexes	319	444 228	218	277 171	192	244 150	171	200 146	100	132 74	61	107 31
Males	290	432 186	224	305 160	224	296 166	166	202 136	100	144 67	33	77 11
Females	349	565 200	205	301 134	140	211 88	156	206 116	100	151 63	96	198 38
Intestinal type												
Both sexes	348	595 185	147	251 78	150	243 86	164	223 117	100	168 55	53	154 11
Males	442	870 190	301	527 156	250	437 129	237	339 160	100	218 37	36	200 9
Females	274	638 88	21	117 5	70	179 19	70	129 33	100	197 43	70	253 8
Diffuse type												
Both sexes	300	876 62	397	730 190	325	598 156	241	386 140	100	256 27	64	356 16
Males	178	643 21	225	490 83	181	395 66	117	215 56	100	256 27	*	
Females	-		-		-		-		*		-	
Number of cases	40		69		74		153		51		12	

* Less than 3 cases.

Table 3. Percentage of Specimens with Intestinal Metaplasia of Stomach in Residents of Cali aged 15 years and older, by Sex and Birthplace

Birthplace	Total Number of specimens	Percentage with metaplasia	Standard error
Nariño	65	58.4	± 6.1
Upper Magdalena	81	46.9	± 5.5
Cauca	102	56.9	± 4.9
Antioquia, Caldas	229	38.4	± 3.2
Cali	393	19.1	± 2.6
Atlantic and Pacific coasts	47	21.3	± 6.0

Table 3. (continued)

	Males			Females		
Birthplace	Number of specimens	Percentage with metaplasia	Standard error	Number of specimens	Percentage with metaplasia	Standard error
Nariño	47	59.6	± 7.2	18	55.6	± 37.0
Upper Magdalena	53	54.7	± 6.8	28	32.1	± 8.8
Cauca	72	55.6	± 5.9	30	60.0	± 8.9
Antioquia, Caldas	151	41.7	± 4.0	78	32.0	± 5.3
Cali	245	21.2	± 2.6	148	16.9	± 3.1
Atlantic and Pacific coasts	31	12.9	± 6.0	16	37.5	± 3.8

coastal cities have very low rates. In addition, we think that the high-risk population harbors a high prevalence of a gastric lesion which is suspected to be premalignant. All these data are inferred from the studies of the population of Cali, a strong pole of attraction for immigrants.

We are now carrying out more in-depth studies of populations of the high- and the low-risk areas in the hope of getting closer to the etiology of gastric cancer. Our strategy is to aim at the identification of factors associated with intestinal metaplasia or other precancerous conditions by examining populations with drastically different prevalence rates of such lesions. For this purpose we are studying the patients of charity hospitals in the high-risk area of the Southern Mountains (Department of Nariño, City of Pasto) and the low-risk area of the Atlantic Coast (Department of Bolivar, City of Cartagena). This part of the study is performed with patients presenting at the hospital for reasons totally unrelated to gastric pathology. A total of 55 patients from the high-risk area of Nariño and Cauca, 30 patients from the department of Bolivar, city of Cartagena, in the low-risk area of the Caribean coast, and 57 natives of Cali have been examined. A special questionnaire directed at discovering signs and symptoms of gastric disease was administered, followed by biochemical tests, gastroacidogram, gastroscopy and gastric biopsy. Fig. 3 shows the prevalence of gastric symptoms in both populations, the symptoms showing the greatest discrimination between the 2 populations are sensations of "fullness" and "heaviness" in the epigastric area, as well as vomiting, nausea, pyrosis and pain. When these symtoms are studied in the light of gastric biopsy findings, as shown in Fig. 4, we see that most of them discriminate between presence or absence of intestinal metaplasia. Fullness and heaviness and, to a lesser extent, gastric pain are good discriminators. They appear to indicate greater bulk of meals or relaxation of the muscular tone. The frequency of pyrosis is interesting since it was found in patients with low gastric acidity. It probably means that in these patients substances other than excessive acid are responsible for this peculiar "heart-burn" sensation. Nausea and a "sour belching" were also found more frequently in patients with intestinal metaplasia. The latter is probably related to fermentation due to low acidity.

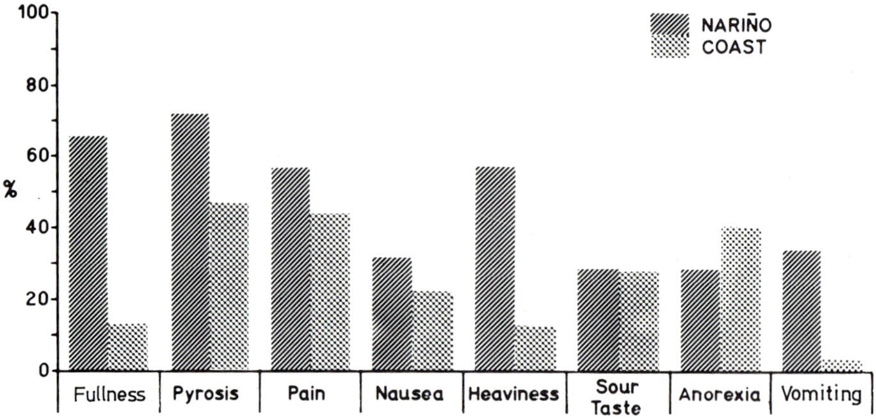

Fig. 3. Percentage of patients with symptoms attributable to gastric pathology. Patients consulting for non-gastric conditions to hospitals of high- (Nariño) and low-risk (coast) areas

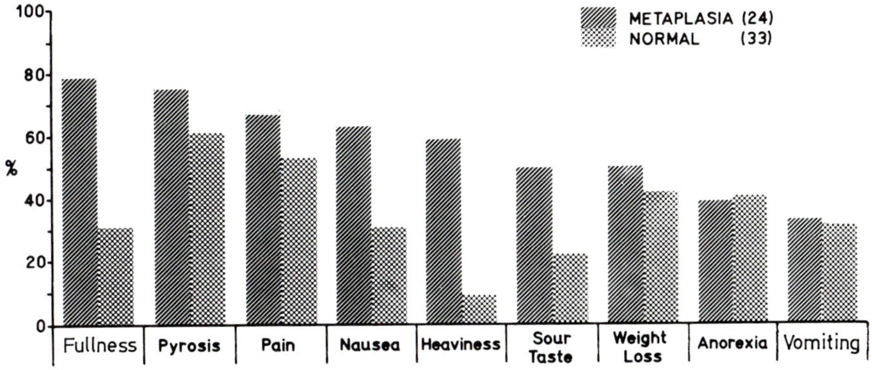

Fig. 4. Percent of patients with symptoms attributable to gastric pathology according to the presence or absence of intestinal metaplasia in gastric biopsies

Table 4. Findings in Gastric Biopsies in Patients admitted to Hospitals for Non-Gastric Conditions

Number of cases	Percent with lesions			
	Normal	Chronic gastritis	Atrophic gastritis	Intestinal metaplasia
Coast	70.0	16.7	6.7	6.7
Valle	45.6	29.8	17.5	7.0
Nariño-Cauca	18.2	12.7	29.1	40.0

Gastric biopsies were taken in these patients. Table 4 shows the results. A much greater prevalence of lesions was found in the high-risk than in the low-risk areas. This was especially true of the more advanced lesions of atrophic gastritis and intestinal metaplasia. Chronic superficial gastritis without atrophy is a fairly common and apparently unspecific finding. Fig. 5 shows the normal gastric mucosa from the body region. Few leukocytes are observed in the lamina propia, and the gastric glands are normal. Fig. 6 is an example of chronic gastritis without atrophy; it shows focal necrosis of the glandular necks. Figs. 7 and 8 are examples of atrophic gastritis and show loss of glands, leukocytic infiltration, and elongation of glandular necks. The number of mitoses is higher in atrophic gastritis with epithelial regeneration. Table 5 shows the prevalence of these lesions in the several populations. Fig. 9 shows an example of intestinal metaplasia in a gastric biopsy. Fig. 10 shows the prevalence of intestinal metaplasia in patients from high- and low-risk areas at different ages. Most of the biochemical tests did not provide any discrimination between the cases of intestinal metaplasia and the persons free of such lesions, although more work needs to be done in this area. Table 6 shows the findings with respect to gastric acidity. Intestinal metaplasia is associated with subnormal acidity.

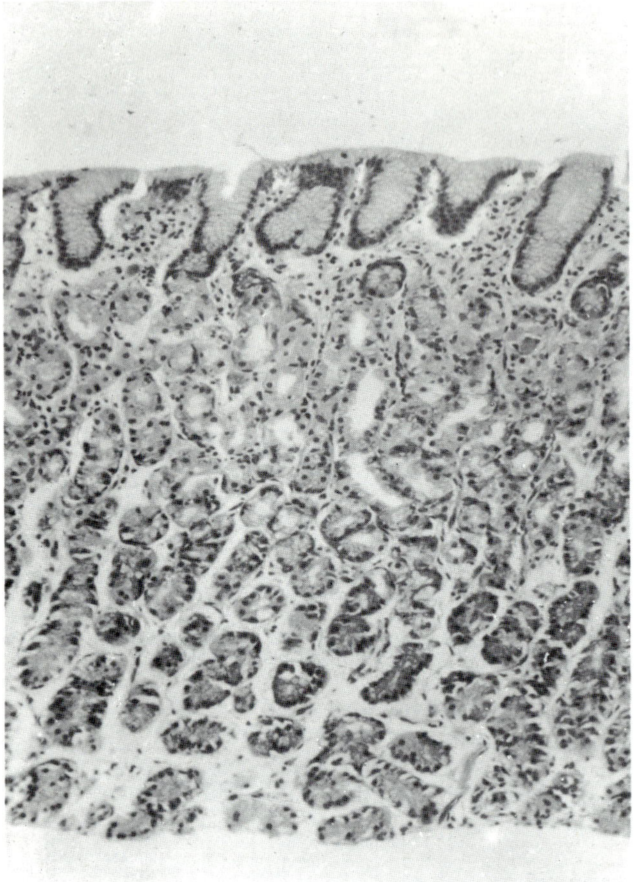

Fig. 5. Normal mucosa. Biopsy from the gastric body

Table 5. Prevalence of Necrosis and Average Number of Mitosis in Glandular Necks

	Bolivar	Valle	Nariño-Cauca
Number of cases	30	101	55
Percentage with necrosis	16.7	49.5	69.1
Average number of mitoses	1.8	3.0	4.4

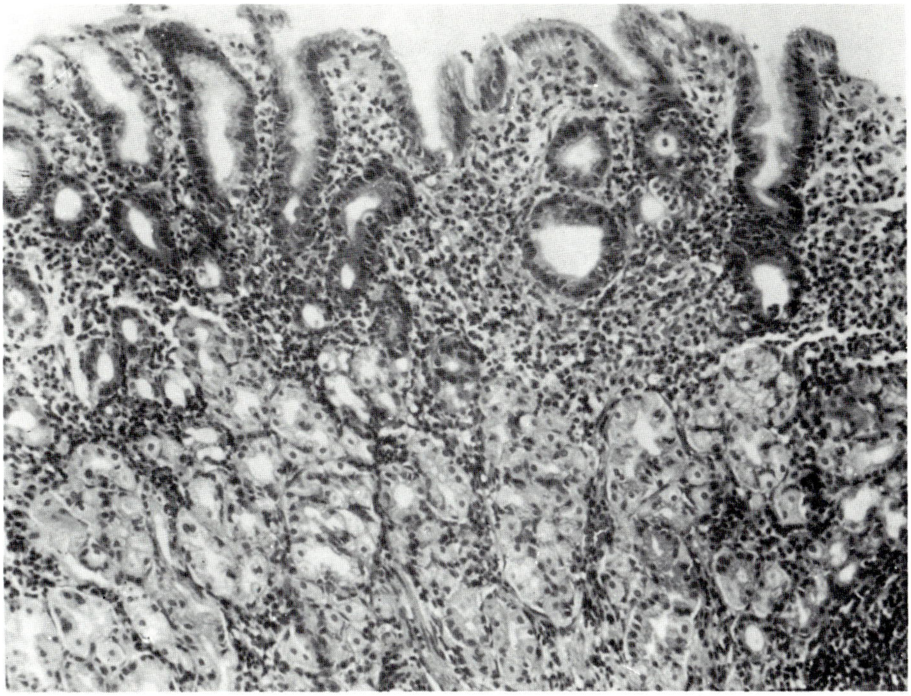

Fig. 6. Gastritis without atrophy. There is superficial infiltration, focal necrosis, and some hyperplasia of the neck region of the glands

Table 6. Gastric Acid in Intestinal Metaplasia

	Patients Normal	$\bar{X}$	Range
Basal	1.7-4.3	0.7	0- 4.4
After stimulation	4.3-22	2.2	0-11.3

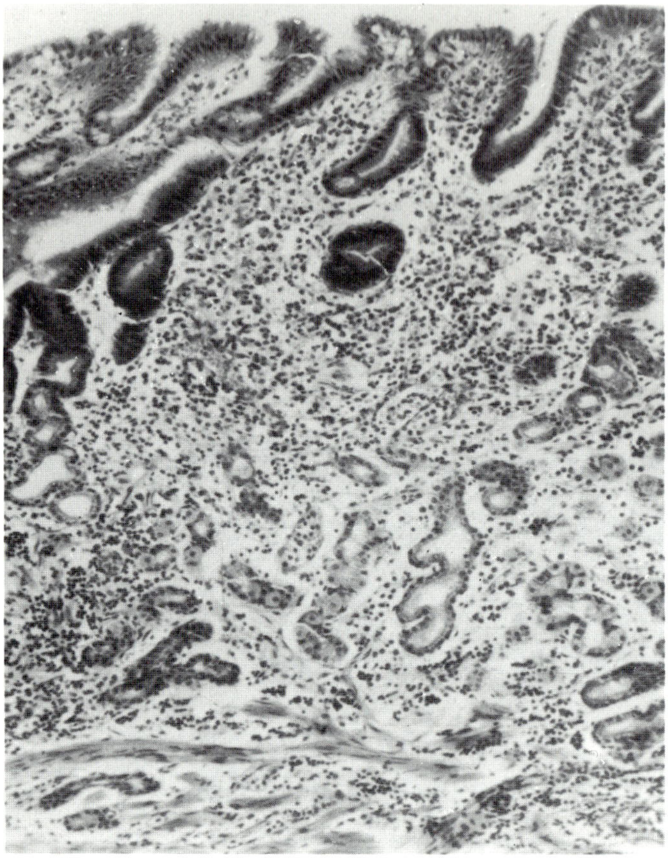

Fig. 7. Atrophic gastritis showing necrosis and loss of glands, leukocytic infiltration, and hyperplasia of the necks of the glands

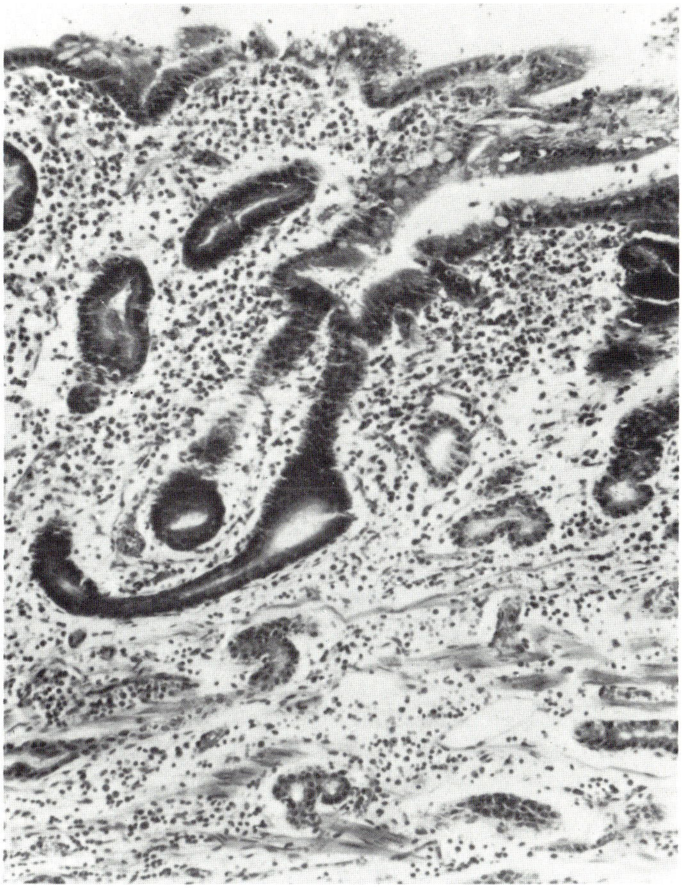

Fig. 8. A more advanced stage of atrophic gastritis, showing marked elongation and hyperplasia of the necks of the glands

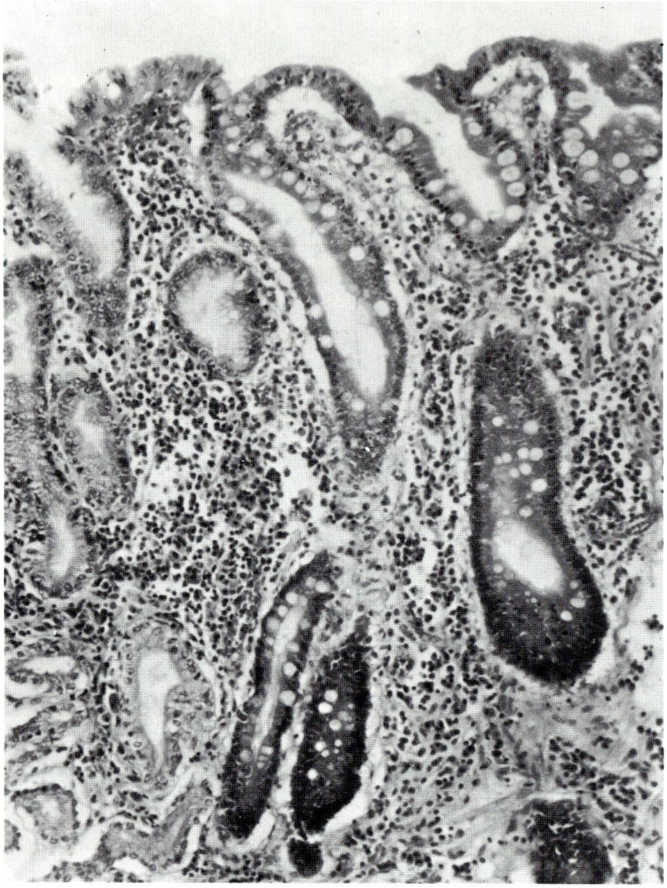

Fig. 9. Atrophic gastritis with intestinal metaplasia

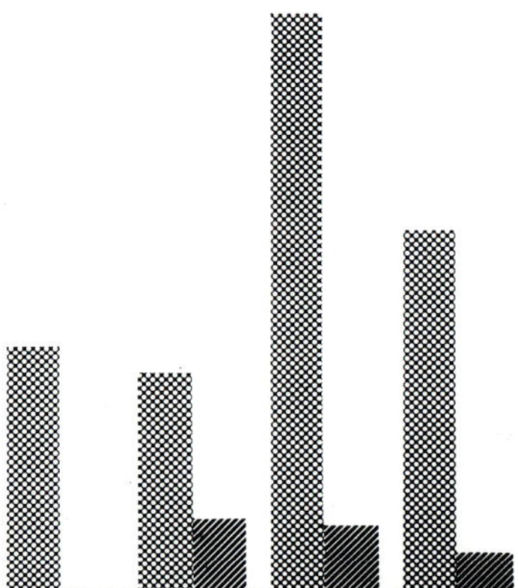

NARIÑO	37.5	33.3	88.8	55.5
COAST	0	11.1	10.0	6.2
AGE ⟶	14-34	35-54	55+	TOTAL

Fig. 10. Prevalence of intestinal metaplasia in gastric biopsies from patients admitted for non-gastric conditions to hospitals of areas of Colombia that are high- (Nariño) and low-risk (coast) for gastric cancer

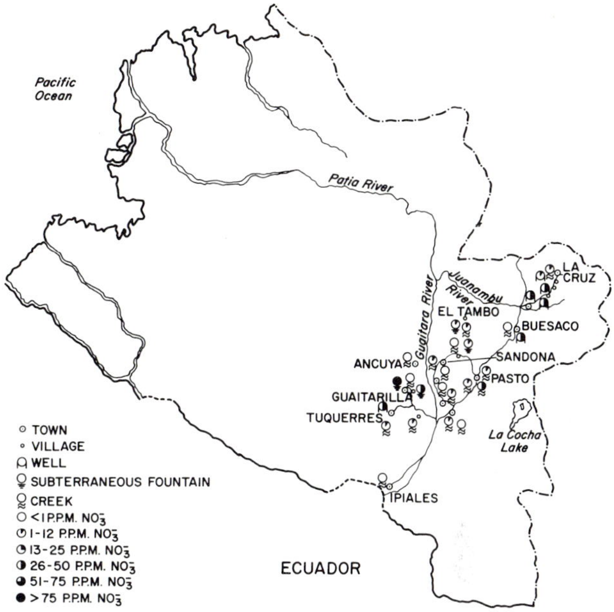

Fig. 11. Map of the department of Narino, showing the findings with respect to nitrate content of water samples

Finally, some limited environmental studies are under way. One of them has to do with the nitrate content of the drinking water. Fig. 11 is a map of the department of Nariño showing a summary of our preliminary findings with respect to the nitrate content of the water supplies. The map shows that in the three areas considered of highest risk for gastric cancer, namely La Cruz, Pasto and Guaitarilla, the water supplies have a high nitrate content. It also shows that dug-wells and subterraneous fountains have higher nitrate concentrations than streams.

References

1. UICC: Cancer Incidence in Five Continents, Vol. II. Eds. DOLL, R., MUIR, C., WATERHOUSE, J. Geneva: UICC 1970.
2. WEBER, I., NARVAEZ, A.: Proyecto demografico del Valle. University of Florida and Universidad del Valle. Unpublished data.
3. JARVI, O., LAUREN, P.: On the role of heterotopias of the intestinal epithelium in the pathogenesis of gastric cancer. Acta path. microbiol. scand. 29, 26 (1951).
4. LAUREN, P.: The two histological main types of gastric carcinoma: Diffuse and so-called intestinal-type carcinoma. An attempt at a histo-clinical classification. Acta path. microbiol. scand. 64, 31 (1965).

The Persistance of Differences in Cancer Incidence at Various Anatomical Sites 1300 Years after Immigration

D. J. Jussawalla

Greater Bombay is a cosmopolitan city with a current population of approximately 6,000,000 persons drawn in sizeable numbers from every State in the Indian Union. This urban centre is thus representative of a true cross-section of the heterogeneous peoples of the country. Thinly dispersed in this vast metropolis, a tiny community known as the Parsis has made significant contribution far beyond what its small numbers would seem to warrant to this city's status as the "Urbs prima in India" (2). The Parsis are distinguished by religious, demographic and socio-economic factors, and even though living in the same geographical environment, present striking differences from other Bombayites in the relative frequency with which cancer is noted at various sites. A critical appraisal of this situation was thus considered promising, in order to ascertain whether or not these apparent differences could be ascribed to recognizable variations in the habits, customs and socio-economic conditions of these people. With this aim in view, we have attempted to investigate the site patterns of risk in this small community in Greater Bombay where the majority of members live, and if possible to define the magnitude and nature of the variations observed.

Historical Background of the Parsis

The Parsis are in fact the sole surviving group of Persian Zoroastrians, who fled their homeland to escape religious persecution during successive waves of invasion by Moslem hoardes, which finally overpowered the weakened Persian Empire by the middle of the seventh century A.D., after 200 years of strife. Refugees wandered away from Persia in various directions and in large numbers, over almost a century, but only small groups who migrated southward are known gradually to have settled along the west coast of India. What happened to the rest remains a mystery. In pursuit of a better life, the Parsis later moved further south again (about 300 years ago), leaving their early rural enclaves along the Gujarat coast in Western India and finally settling in Bombay City in large numbers.

The community is highly inbred, and fully two-thirds of its members, out of a total world population of 120,000, reside within the Greater Bombay area. The economic status, literacy rate and various habits and customs of these people appear to be at variance with those of other communities in the City. This small group is unusually enlightened, enterprising, economically prosperous and westernized (2, 8).

All through the years, the Parsis maintained cordial relations with other local communities, but to preserve their solidarity and existence as a community, rigid norms of social and religious behaviour were prescribed and followed. As a general rule, the Parsis are required to refrain from smoking on religious grounds, marriages are undertaken almost exclusively within the communal fold and proselytization, the conversion of non-Parsis to the Zoroastrian faith, is also totally prohibited. Zoroastrianism was founded over 3000 years ago as one of the earliest monotheistic religions of the world after Judaism.

Area and Population of Greater Bombay

This survey, undertaken by the Bombay Cancer Registry, has been strictly restricted to the residents of Greater Bombay, a densely populated urban centre on the West coast of India, occupying an area of 437.7 km^2.

The population figures used to compute the incidence rates have been interpolated from the projected population of Greater Bombay (3). Only cancer patients confirmed as having been resident in Bombay for a minimum of 1 year have been included in this study.

Special tables based on the 1961 data and giving the age composition of the Parsi population were obtained and used to estimate the age distribution (1).

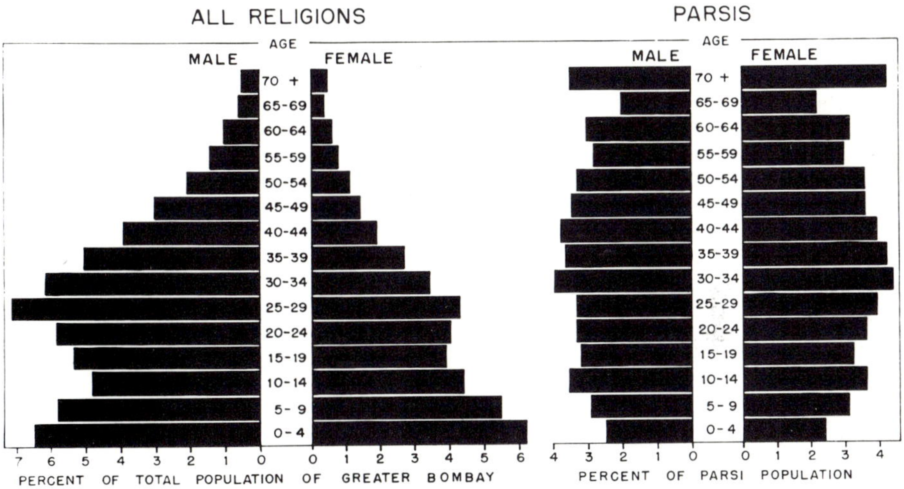

Fig. 1. Population for Parsis and all religions, Greater Bombay, 1964-1966

The Parsis account for only 1.7 percent of the total number of residents of Greater Bombay, and present an age pyramid remarkably different from that of the population of the city as a whole (Fig. 1).

Differences in the age composition, habits, customs and ethnic characteristics have all provided important leads for the study of cancer in this small community. It is a sign of the times that some of the religious and social customs which were rigidly upheld by the older generations are rapidly giving way to "modernism", and it is felt that in the foreseeable future the characteristic identity of this community may be lost for ever.

Incidence Rates

In the United States, a vast amount of effort seems to have been devoted to the study of cancer rates and ratios in its white and non-white populations. These studies have revealed significant differences in the prevalence and incidence of cancer between these two ethnic groups and have proved useful in elucidating a number of etiological factors responsible for the occurrence of cancer at specific sites. There have, however, been very few inquiries elsewhere to estimate differences in cancer risks between ethnic subgroups and between various religious sects living together in one geographical area (7).

We have attempted to examine the cancer incidence rates at various anatomical sites in the different religious groups residing in Greater Bombay, in order to identify any variations present. Although the residents of Bombay belong to a number of differing religious sects, data obtained from the whole metropolitan area tend to reflect predominantly the Hindu experience, because of the overwhelming majority of these people in the general population. The individual Hindu, Muslim and Christian contrasts are beyond the scope of this presentation, which has been restricted to the differences found in site-specific cancer risks between the Parsis and the total Bombay population.

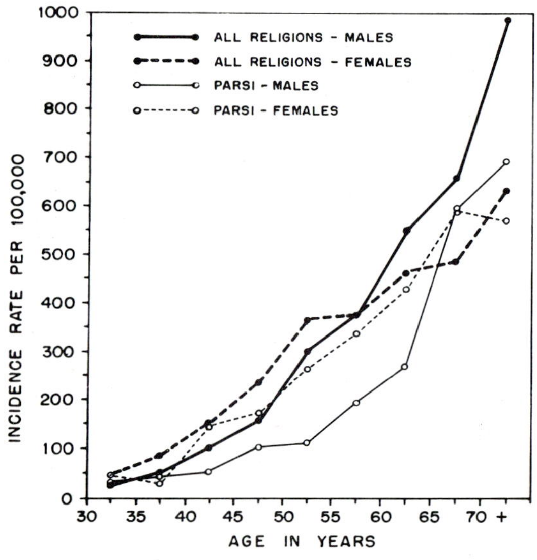

Fig. 2. Age-specific cancer incidence rates per 100,000 population for all religions & Parsis, Greater Bombay, 1964-1966

The sex and age-specific incidence rates for the Parsi residents and for the total population of Greater Bombay are shown in Fig. 2.

The variations in age-specific incidence rates are due to the smallness of the sample in some of the age groups, but on the whole, incidence rates tend to follow the general pattern of increase with age, for both the populations studied.

Age-Adjusted Rates

For adequate comparison, all cancer incidence rates have been adjusted to the world standard population, as suggested by Doll (9). Such adjusted rates computed for the Parsi community and for the Bombay population taken as a whole are compared with the reported data from Norway, 1959-61, and England and Wales (4 regions), 1960-62 (9).

The male preponderance observed in various registers is also seen in Greater Bombay, but the Parsis surprisingly present a reverse pattern.

The over-all age-adjusted rates for Greater Bombay (all religions), though low, are not the lowest reported in the literature (4). For some, as yet unknown, reason, the Parsis present even lower rates, only two African registers, in Nigeria (Ibadan) and Uganda (Kyadondo), having recorded lower rates.

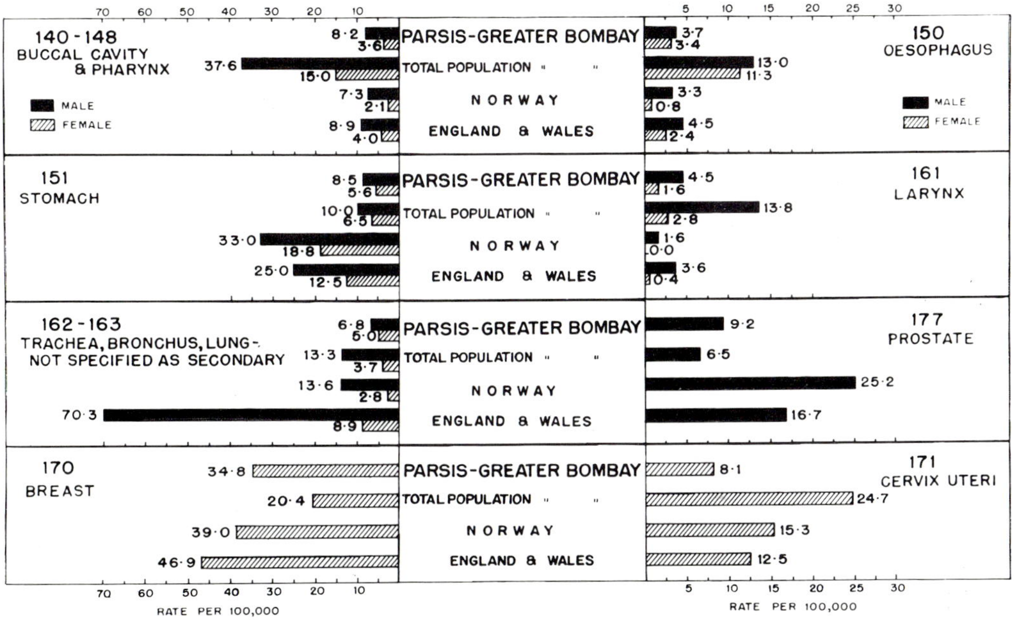

Fig. 3. Age-adjusted rates at selected sites for the Parsis in Greater Bombay, compared with the rates for total Bombay population 1964-1966, Norway 1959-1961 and England & Wales 1960-1962

Certain specific sites are less commonly affected by cancer in the Parsis than in the total Bombay population. These sites are the buccal cavity, pharynx, larynx, oesophagus and cervix uteri (Fig. 3). On the other hand, the Parsi rates are higher for a number of other sites, such as the pancreas, prostate, bladder, nervous system, female breast, body of the uterus and ovary, and there is also a higher incidence of leukaemias in this community.

It is interesting to note that specific sub-sites within the boundaries of the buccal cavity and pharynx, which are frequently affected by cancer in the Greater Bombay population as a whole, are not attended by similarly high risks in the Parsis. Thus, for example, cancer of the oesophagus, which is 5th in order of frequency in males and 3rd in females in Greater Bombay is 8th on the list (in both sexes) in the Parsi community.

The prostate, in contrast, which is the commonest site for cancer in Parsi men, ranks only 7th in the total city population. Similarly, the female breast, the leading cancer site in Parsi women, changes place with the uterine cervix as the commonest target in all the other religious groups. Thus, the Parsi pattern appears to differ radically from that of Greater Bombay as a whole.

Observations on Cancer Affecting Selected Major Anatomical Regions: Oral Cavity and Pharynx

In Greater Bombay, the oral cavity and pharynx are the most frequent sites of malignant tumours and display very high age-adjusted rates, in contrast to the situation observed in other countries throughout the world (4). The Parsis of Bombay, however, present much lower incidence rates for both these anatomical areas.

But the Parsis and the total Bombay population both reveal a higher incidence of oral (Int. List No. 140-144) than pharyngeal cancer (Int. List No. 145, 147-148).

In the oral and pharyngeal regions, the tongue is the most common subsite in Parsi men, and the buccal mucosa and other parts of the mouth (Int. List No. 144) in Parsi women. However, none of these cancers even approaches the ten leading sites in this community in frequency.

Male preponderance is dominant in this anatomical region amongst all residents of Bombay, including the Parsis.

Age-adjusted rates for cancers of the buccal cavity and pharynx in the Parsis are comparable to the British and Norwegian figures but show some variations in the site-specific rates.

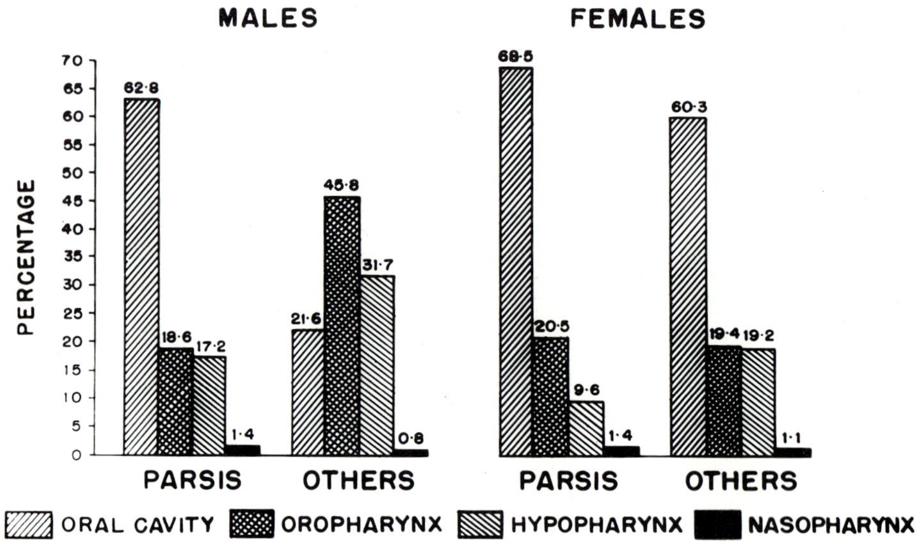

Fig. 4

The majority of cancer patients in Bombay are seen and treated at the Tata Memorial Hospital, and data from this Hospital also show that the frequency ratios for cancer in the oral and pharyngeal regions, which are high in the Hindus and Muslims, seem to be of minimal importance in the Parsis. (The distribution of cancer within the oral and pharyngeal regions in this community is shown in Fig. 4.) It is obvious that in this group, when cancer does occur in this region, it affects the oral cavity more often than the pharynx, and within the oral cavity the anterior two-thirds of the tongue is the favoured sub-site, another contrast with the total Bombay experience.

The low Parsi rates for oral and pharyngeal cancers are perhaps related to the fact that this group is less addicted to smoking and almost totally abstains from chewing tobacco. These habits are very prevalent in the other communities, which are known to present higher rates at these sites.

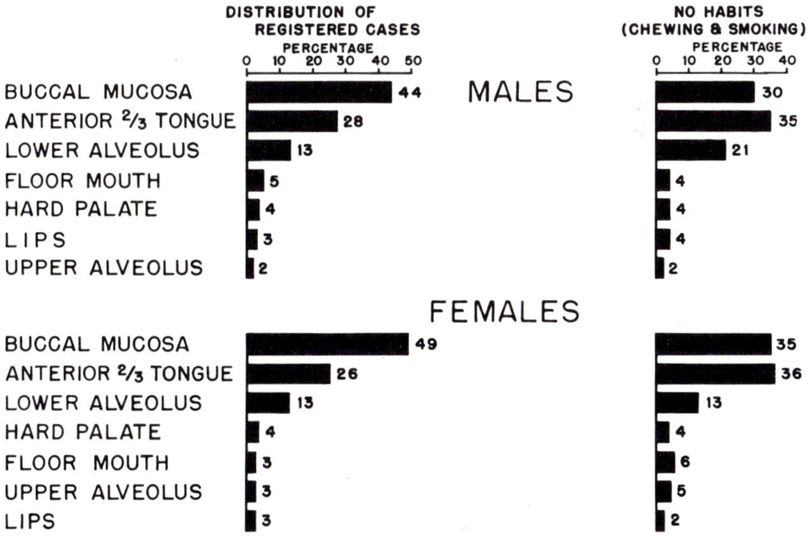

Fig. 5

In those who have no fixed habits, the distribution of cancer within the oral cavity shows slight deviations from the total experience, the anterior two-thirds of the tongue showing a higher incidence than the buccal mucosa (Fig. 5). The Parsis present a pattern similar to those who have no addiction to smoking or tobacco chewing.

The Digestive Organs

In Greater Bombay, the oesophagus is clearly the viscus most favoured by cancer in the gastro-intestinal tract, with age-adjusted rates about the 9th highest recorded in world literature (6). At this site again, the risk among Parsis (both sexes) is much lower, the male rate being similar to that observed in Norway and somewhat lower than that in England and Wales. Parsi women, however, show a comparatively higher incidence of cancer at this site than British and Norwegian members of their own sex.

One of the prominent epidemiological characteristics of oesophageal cancer is the wide variation seen in the sex ratio in different geographical areas of the world. The greater Bombay population, including the Parsis, presents low M : F ratios at this site. The reason for this unusual, near-equal sex incidence is not yet clear, and may indicate a common environmental or dietary aetiology in the two sexes.

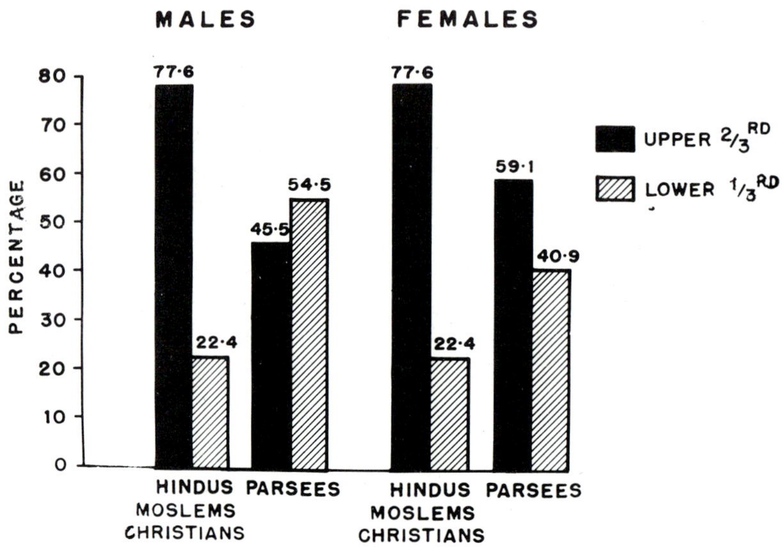

Fig. 6

The regional distribution of cancer over the whole length of the oesophagus was also seen to vary between the two groups. In the Tata Hospital series, the lower third of the oesophagus is involved more often in the Parsis, in contrast to the upper two-thirds in other communities (Fig. 6). In this community, 13 percent of cancers of the lower third of the oesophagus were adenocarcinomas, more or less the same as the 11 percent in the rest. In fact, the investigation for any connexion with specific habits seems to indicate a strong association of smoking and tobacco chewing with cancer in the upper two-thirds of the thoracic oesophagus rather than in the lower third in our patients.

The total Bombay population proves to be low-risk for cancers of the stomach, colon and rectum (4), risks among the Parsis being the same or lower (Fig. 7).

The ratio of the incidence of stomach to oesophageal cancer usually favours the former site in most countries. The values recorded for Parsis in Bombay follow this universal rule, in contrast to the total Bombay population in which the pattern is reversed.

Throughout the world there is a preponderance of intestinal cancer in women (Int. List No. 152-153). Greater Bombay, however, has an atypical sex ratio with a much higher incidence in men. The Parsis lean towards the international pattern in this condition also.

The male predominance in cases of cancer of the stomach and rectum also holds true for the total Bombay population, including the Parsi group.

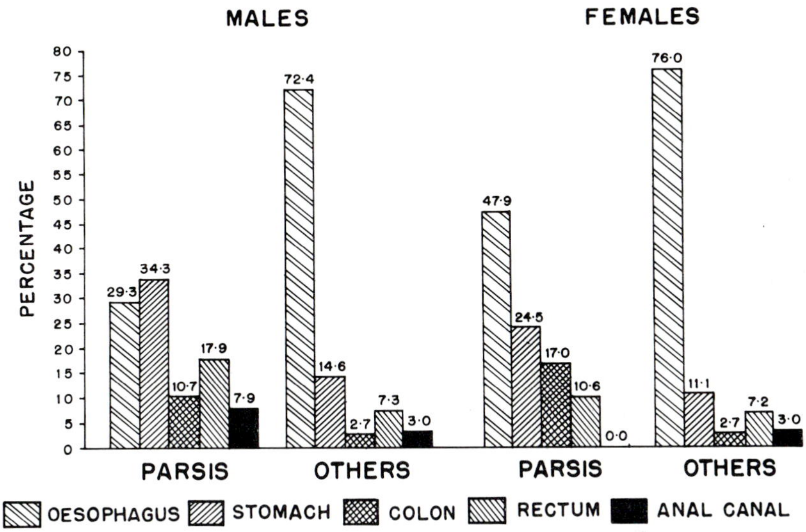

Fig. 7

This small community, however, has a higher incidence of pancreatic cancer, in contrast to the total Bombay population, although the Parsi figures are still somewhat lower than Norwegian and British rates.

Respiratory System

The age-adjusted rates for laryngeal cancer in Greater Bombay are the highest in any country, being 50 percent higher than the figure reported from Jamaica, which comes next in rank (4). Even at this high-risk site in Bombay, the Parsis seem to present a low profile, although their incidence rate for this site is somewhat higher than that of the British and Norwegian populations.

Cancer of the bronchus or lung (not specified as secondary) is relatively infrequent in Greater Bombay (4). Parsi men confirm to this pattern, revealing even lower comparative rates, but Parsi women present somewhat higher incidence rates than the overall group of Bombay females.

The ratio of lung to larynx cancer is greatly in favour of the former site in almost all countries throughout the world. The Parsis follow this standard pattern, but once again, in Greater Bombay males the pattern is reversed.

Cancer of the Female Breast

At the Tata Memorial Hospital, almost 51 percent of all cancers in women are seen in the breast in the Parsi group, in contrast to the lesser ratio of 25 percent observed in the other communities (excepting the Moslem women), in whom cancer of the cervix is the most common form (Fig. 8).

This high frequency of female breast cancer in the Parsis has attracted our attention for the past decade, and with the data obtained from the Bombay Cancer Registry, a somewhat clearer picture of the situation has now emerged.

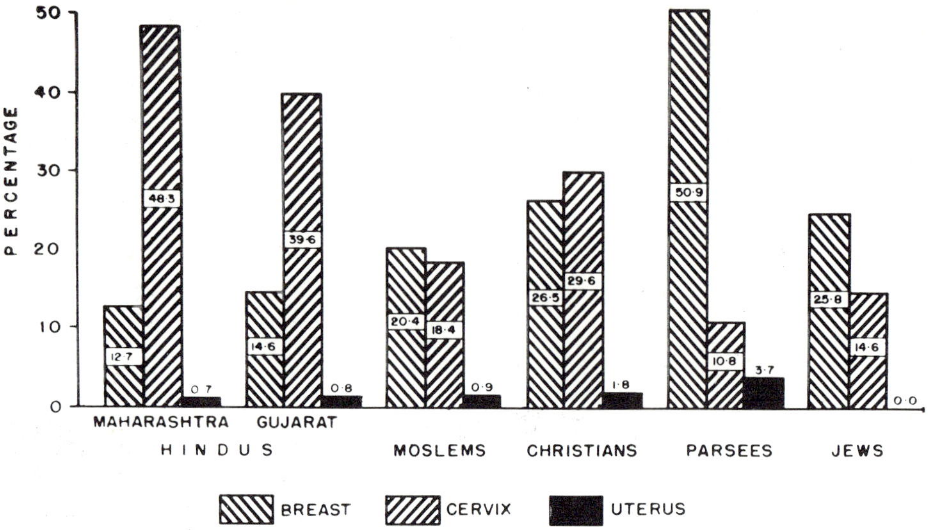

Fig. 8

The breast is the second commonest site affected by cancer in Bombay females, but is the most common site in Parsi women, just as it is in Norway, England, and other Western countries. In comparison with Western data, the overall age-adjusted rates are also lower in Greater Bombay (4). In Parsi women, however, adjusted rates are 1.7 times higher than in the total number of Bombay women, but they are still lower than the Norwegian and English figures.

The social factors that may have a bearing on the high incidence of cancer of the breast in Parsi women are: late marriage, infrequent breast feeding and low fertility rate. More Parsi women seem to remain unmarried than those of the other communities. The average age at marriage is also comparatively higher in the Parsi group. Investigations at the Tata Centre have also shown that a particle similar to the c particle implicated as the milk factor in spontaneous breast cancer of mice has been seen with disturbing frequency in the milk of Parsi mothers.

Cancer of the Female Genital Tract

The cervix is the commonest cancer site in Bombay women. It assumes an intermediate rank on international comparison (4). Here again in Parsi women the rate is only one third that recorded for the total female population of Bombay, an even lower incidence than in Norway or Britain.

Cancer of the corpus uteri, in contrast, is commonly seen in Parsi females, its incidence being more than twice that observed in all Bombay women taken together. In British and Norwegian women, however, the incidence is even higher than in the Parsis.

All registers which reveal high adjusted rates for cervical cancer also present a high cervix-to-corpus ratio. Greater Bombay follows the universal pattern, which is in direct contrast to that among the Parsis, which appears to follow the universal rule of "low rates and lower ratios". The high cervix-to-corpus ratio in Greater Bombay in fact reflects the low corpus rates rather than high cervix rates.

Cancers involving the ovaries, Fallopian tubes and broad ligament are second in incidence in Parsi women, although the age-adjusted rates are lower than those reported from Norway and from England and Wales.

Cancer of the Male Genital Organs

The Parsi rates for cancers involving the male genital organs (grouped together), are higher than the figures reported for the total Bombay population; but this is entirely due to a high prostate incidence, though Britain and Norway have reported even higher incidences of prostatic cancer.

Analyses of age-specific rates demonstrate that the earliest prostatic lesions are seen between the ages of 40 and 50 in most countries, whereas the highest incidence is noted in the age groups 65-69 and above. The Parsis, with a large segment of their population in the older age groups, thus seem to present a higher incidence than the total male population of Bombay.

Other Sites

Comparison of age-adjusted rates for other sites with the corresponding data from Norway and England and Wales does not reveal anything of significance.

The overall incidence of skin cancer is very low in Greater Bombay. Here again the Parsis have an incidence over 150 percent that attained by the total Bombay population, although the incidence at this site is also much lower than that in England and Wales.

The frequency ratio of skin cancer in the Tata Hospital series is also relatively higher for the Parsi community. A comparison of various histological types of skin cancer seen in the different communities shows that basal cell cancer is most common in the Parsis, and such a pattern is otherwise seen only amongst foreigners resident in Bombay (mostly from Western countries) (Fig. 9). In the other local religious groups, squamous cell carcinomas far outnumber the basal cell variety. The high prevalence of basal cell cancer in the Parsis is probably due to their lighter skin pigmentation and lesser exposure to the causal factors which increase the risk of squamous cell carcinomas, particularly in the region of the trunk and lower extremities.

Leukaemia is also common in this small community, and its incidence appears to be higher than in the British but lower than in the Norwegians.

Conclusion and Comments

The high incidence of cancer of the breats in Parsi women and of the prostate in Parsi men has long claimed our attention. In fact, reports from individual hospitals also confirm this situation. It is thought that these different site patterns may be due to the variations observed in the habits, customs and economic status of this small group. Speculative explanations for the high risk for certain sites in the

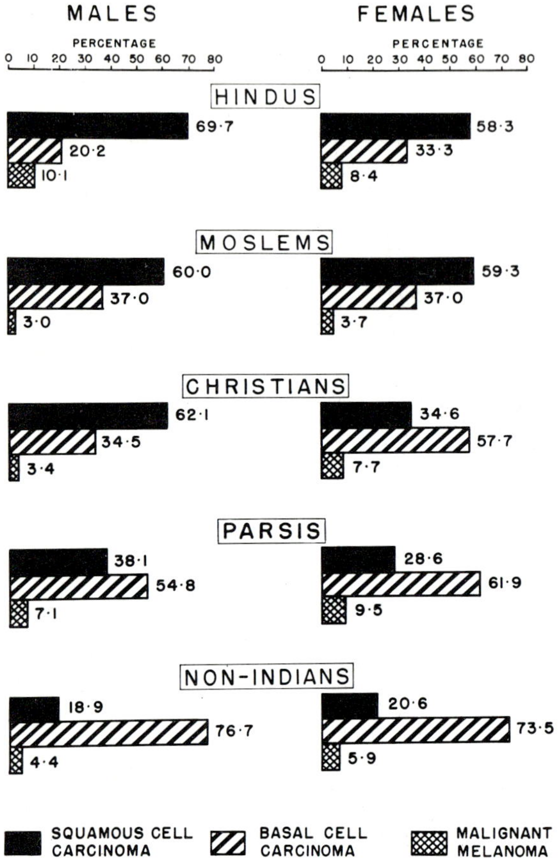

Fig. 9

Parsis include late marriage, infrequent breast feeding and a low fertility rate. Moderate smoking and minimal tobacco chewing, in association with a relatively high socio-economic status and westernized dietary and living habits and a different pattern of the age pyramid are other factors found to be at variance with the situation observed in other communities living in Bombay. The presence in the breast milk of Parsi women of particles similar to the c particle that is believed to be the Bittner milk factor, which is found in breast-cancer-prone mice, is another disturbing finding.

A previous report by other workers on the Parsi experience was based on relative frequency ratios obtained from an individual hospital data bank, and at one time it was also suspected that the differences noted in the frequency ratios of cancer at specific sites between the Parsis and the other communities might be due to the different age structure of the Parsi population. Surprisingly, however, we find that although the differences in incidence rates of a variety of cancers do indeed narrow down on age-adjustment, the reversal of site pattern seems to persist.

In the absence of any convincing evidence to the importance of major genetic factors in the aetiology of cancer, it does not seem likely that they play any significant role in the observed differences in the site incidence of cancer amongst various communities living side by side in a given geographical area. The exact significance of the frequent presence of 'c'-like particles in the breastmilk is not yet clear. It appears more realistic to conjecture that differences noted in the various environmental factors, personal habits and communal customs of the different sections of a population might explain some of the variations observed in the relative cancer risks.

In order to identify the aetiological factors that might be implicated in a segment of a selected population, such as that of Bombay, case-control studies of the Parsi community with its unusual risk patterns at certain sites are already under way. This project should be helpful in establishing the differences, if any, in a number of suspect factors, such as age at marriage, breast-feeding habits, number of pregnancies, tobacco-smoking and -chewing habits, type and quality of food ingested, standard of nutrition, personal hygiene, economic status, etc. The Parsis, luckily, happen to be concentrated in the Greater Bombay area, and this investigation should be completed in the foreseeable future.

References

1. Census of India: Parsis of Greater Bombay, Vol. X, Maharashtra, part X(1-D) Bombay: Government Central Press 1961.
2. CHANDRASEKAR, C.: (1948), Human Biology 20, 47 (1948).
3. Bombay Municipal Corporation: Development plan for Greater Bombay. Bombay: Government Central Press 1948.
4. JUSSAWALLA, D. J., HAENSZEL, W., DESHPANDE, V. A., NATEKAR, M. V.: Brit. J. Cancer 22, 623 (1968).
5. JUSSAWALLA, D. J., HAENSZEL, W., DESHPANDE, V. A., NATEKAR, M. V.: Brit. J. Cancer 24, 56 (1970).
6. JUSSAWALLA, D. J.: Int. J. Cancer 10, 436 (1972).
7. MACMAHON, B.: Acta Un. Int. Cancer 16, 1716 (1960).
8. RELE, J. R.: Brit. J. prev. soc. Med. 14, 181 (1960).
9. UICC: Cancer Incidence in Five Continents, Vols 1 and 2. Berlin: Springer 1966, 1970.

Closing Remarks

The Future of Cancer Registries

E. Pedersen

Although cancer registration was initiated in several countries early in this century, the great majority of registries currently in existence have been established since 1950. The rapid development during the 'fifties can be attributed to the striking results achieved by a few registries established during the preceding 20 years in Denmark, Great Britain and the United States of America. Their work gradually made it apparent that modern society cannot do without data of crucial importance in the investigation of major causes of disability and death or in the planning and evaluation of extremely costly medical services. We have since seen increasing activity and productivity of cancer registries. Several registries will recall with gratitude the impetus and guidance provided by institutions such as the US National Cancer Institute and, more recently, the International Agency for Research on Cancer in Lyons. Both have initiated and stimulated cancer registration - ad hoc or for general purposes - in several regions and have raised a number of registries to a level of efficiency which they could otherwise hardly have attained.

In recent years, increasing numbers of cancer registries have successfully switched to automated data processing, and these have probably all found that their analytic potential has been greatly increased. Judging from experience in Norway, the problem now is not so much how to explore and analyze the data technically, but how to assign priorities. The pressure of interesting and important problems that are deserving of investigation seems to be inreasing all the time. Current problems will keep us busy for many years to come, and new problems will doubtless present themselves and require our attention at a tempo not paralleled by our working capacity.

Increasing computerization of medical data may create some future problems for cancer registries. Several countries are contemplating, or actually testing, systems requiring submission to some central data bank of information on all hospitalized persons, regardless of diagnosis. There is some concern that once such a system is adopted it may be impossible to continue cancer registration as a separate process. Should it be decided to maintain the cancer registry for analytical purposes, it would have to draw the data from the central bank, and it is generally felt that these data will be of inferior quality to those obtained by independent registration of cancer cases.

For the comprehensive disease registration suggested above to be useful, a very large staff would be required for data analysis. It is conceivable that some cancer registries may gradually develop into, or become absorbed by, larger statistical/epidemiological institutions responsible for the analysis of a wide range of medical data.

At this Symposium we have repeatedly returned to the problem of data protection, and we have all been struck by the highly dissimilar ways in which different countries - even within Europe - are dealing with this problem. While in some central European countries professional discretion virtually precludes meaningful cancer registration, in others the introduction of comprehensive registration, with complete identification of persons, has stirred little or no public debate. However, even in these countries, with the increasing tendency to centralized computerization of medical data there are growing signs of concern over inadequate protection of data relating to persons. The future consequences of this apparent change of attitude are difficult to foresee. In some countries (e.g. in Scandinavia), where the cancer registry is regarded as an essential instrument in the fight against cancer, it is unlikely that there will be any restrictions on reporting to the registry or on the usage of data by the registry.

As emphasized above, in the foreseeable future cancer registries will be faced with more challenging problems than they can adequately handle. Thus the allocation of priorities will have to continue. In order to avoid wastage or obsolescence of highly important registry data, however, cooperation should be invited from other interested and competent parties to ensure the fullest possible utilization of the material. For example, clinical departments should be encouraged to undertake periodic survival studies and should be offered any necessary assistance. We have been doing this for some time in Norway, and hospitals are submitting lists of patients with requests for information about their survival status with increasing frequency. A list can generally be returned within one day, with information about those who have died, including the time of death and stated cause of death. Assistance in survival analysis is also available. Besides being important in the evaluation of therapy, this form of service also creates goodwill, increases cooperation, and ensures a good quality of reporting from institutions.

Pathologists have also been approached, and we find them increasingly interested in exploring and consulting the national histopathology data bank that we are accumulating. They have found the creation of the bank perfectly acceptable. A rapid increase in the usage of the data for research purposes is foreseen.

It is beyond the scope of this paper to discuss what specific projects should be given priority in the coming years, but there is one field of activity that is likely to become extremely important in the future, i.e. the search for evidence of carcinogenic exposure in occupational groups. For many reasons, such studies have been rare in the past, despite the fact that dangerous exposure is known to exist, or strongly suspected, in many types of occupations. Dr. Waterhouse has given an elegant demonstration of the great potential of the registry for carrying out studies of this nature cheaply and efficiently. A similar study to his (of cancer risk among nickel workers) has recently been completed in Norway, based on methods that have only just become applicable, and the authorities were so impressed by the results and by the smoothness and low cost of the operation, that a program based on the Cancer Registry and amounting to a permanent surveillance of our major industries is now being considered. In preparation for this program record linkage of the entire 1960 census population by occupation against the Registry material for the years 1961-72 and the national mortality data for the same period is to be carried out. Regional analysis is expected to yield at least some indication of the major problem areas. We are also to receive lists of past and current employees from several of our larger industries.

The development going on in this field is highly important. Cancer registries in many countries will find that they are in a unique position to assume a leading role in this type of epidemiological research.

With a view to the future, I should like to recall a very important event in the history of cancer registration, namely the agreement between the International Association of Cancer Registries and the International Agency for Research on Cancer in Lyons. I believe that the future consequences of this will be great, and beneficial to both parties. Many important epidemiological cancer problems can only be adequately investigated if countries cooperate, and international cooperation on projects is one of the major objectives of the agreement. Activity is sure to be greatly increased, and we shall have the benefit of learning from each other. In this context, it seems likely that the International Agency in Lyons will also develop into a training center for epidemiological research. There is clearly a need for such a center in Europe.

In concluding, let me emphasize that our future is going to depend on what we achieve, which will depend on our imagination, incentive and competence, and on the resources and facilities made available to us. These resources will depend in turn on what we achieve.

Subject Index

Recent Results in Cancer Research

Sponsored by the Swiss League against Cancer. Editor in Chief: P. Rentchnick, Genève

1 SCHINDLER, R.: Die tierische Zelle in Zellkultur. Geb. DM 19,80; US $ 8.10

2 Neuroblastomas — Biochemical Studies. Edited by C. BOHUON, (Symposium). Cloth DM 19,80; US $ 8.10

3 HUEPER, W. C.: Occupational and Environmental Cancers of the Respiratory System. Cloth DM 41,00; US $ 16.80

4 GOLDMAN, L.: Laser Cancer Research. Cloth DM 19,80; US $ 8.10

5 METCALF, D.: The Thymus. Its Role in Immune Responses, Leukaemia Development and Carcinogenesis. Cloth DM 29,00; US $ 11.90

6 Malignant Transformation by Viruses. Edited by W. H. KIRSTEN, (Symposium). Cloth DM 39,00; US $ 16.00

7 MOERTEL, CH. G.: Multiple Primary Malignant Neoplasms. Their Incidence and Significance. Cloth DM 22,00; US $ 9.00

8 New Trends in the Treatment of Cancer. Edited by L. MANUILA, S. MOLES, and P. RENTCHNICK. Cloth DM 39,00; US $ 16.00

9 LINDENMANN, J., and P. A. KLEIN: Immunological Aspects of Viral Oncolysis. Cloth DM 22,00; US $ 9.00

10 NELSON, R. S.: Radioactive Phosphorus in the Diagnosis of Gastrointestinal Cancer. Cloth DM 19,00; US $ 7.80

11 FREEMAN, R. G., and J. M. KNOX: Treatment of Skin Cancer. Cloth DM 19,00; US $ 7.80

12 LYNCH, H. T.: Hereditary Factors in Carcinoma. Cloth DM 29,00; US $ 11.90

13 Tumours in Children. Edited by H. B. MARSDEN and J. K. STEWARD. Cloth DM 87,00; US $ 35.50

14 ODARTCHENKO, N.: Production Cellulaire Erythropoiétique. Relié DM 34,00; US $ 13.90

15 SOKOLOFF, B.: Carcinoid and Serotonin. Cloth DM 29,00; US $ 11.90

16 JACOBS, M. L.: Malignant Lymphomas and Their Management. Cloth DM 22,00; US $ 9.00

17 Normal and Malignant Cell Growth. Edited by R. J. M. FRY, M. L. GRIEM, and W. H. KIRSTEN (Symposium). Cloth DM 63,00; US $ 25.70

18 ANGLESIO, E.: The Treatment of Hodgkin's Disease. Cloth DM 26,50; US $ 10.90

19 BANNASCH, P.: The Cytoplasm of Hepatocytes during Carcinogenesis. Electron- and Lightmicroscopical Investigations of the Nitrosomorpholine-intoxicated Rat Liver. Cloth DM 35,50; US $ 14.50

20 Rubidomycin. A new Agent against Cancer. Edited by J. BERNARD, R. PAUL, M. BOIRON, C. JACQUILLAT, and R. MARAL. Cloth DM 53,00; US $ 21.70

21 Scientific Basis of Cancer Chemotherapy. Edited by G. MATHÉ (Symposium). Cloth DM 31,00; US $ 12.70

22 KOLDOVSKÝ, P.: Tumor Specific Transplantation Antigen. Cloth DM 26,50; US $ 10.90

23 FUCHS, W. A., J. W. DAVIDSON, and H. W. FISCHER: Lymphography in Cancer. With contributions by G. JANTET and H. RÖSLER. Cloth DM 84,00; US $ 34.30

24 HAYWARD, J. L.: Hormones and Human Breast Cancer. An Account of 15 Years Study. Cloth DM 37,50; US $ 15.30

25 ROY-BURMAN, P.: Analogues of Nucleic Acid Components. Mechanisms of Action. Cloth DM 31,00; US $ 12.70

26 Tumors of the Liver. Edited by G. T. PACK and A. H. ISLAMI. Cloth DM 62,00; US $ 25.30

27 SZYMENDERA, J.: Bone Mineral Metabolism in Cancer. Cloth DM 35,50; US $ 14.50

28 MEEK, E. S.: Antitumour and Antiviral Substances of Natural Origin. Cloth DM 18,00; US $ 7.40

29 Aseptic Environments and Cancer Treatment. Edited by G. MATHÉ (Symposium). Cloth DM 24,50; US $ 10.00

30 Advances in the Treatment of Acute (Blastic) Leukemias. Edited by G. MATHÉ (Symposium). Cloth DM 42,00; US $ 17.20

31 DENOIX, P.: Treatment of Malignant Breast Tumors. Indications and Results. Cloth DM 53,00; US $ 21.70

32 NELSON, R. S.: Endoscopy in Gastric Cancer. Cloth DM 53,00; US $ 21.70

33 Experimental and Clinical Effects of L-Asparaginase. Edited by E. GRUNDMANN and H. F. OETTGEN (Symposium). Cloth DM 64,00; US $ 26.20

34 Chemistry and Biological Actions of 4-Nitroquinoline 1-Oxide. Edited by H. ENDO, T. ONO, and T. SUGIMURA. Cloth DM 36,—; US $ 14.70

35 PENN, I.: Malignant Tumors in Organ Transplant Recipients. Cloth DM 26,50; US $ 10.90

36 Current Concepts in the Management of Lymphoma and Leukemia. Edited by J. E. ULTMANN, M. L. GRIEM, W. H. KIRSTEN, and R. W. WISSLER (Symposium). Cloth DM 48,—; US $ 19.60

37 CHIAPPA, S., R. MUSUMECI, and C. USLENGHI: Endolymphatic Radiotherapy in Malignant Lymphomas. With contributions by G. BONADONNA, B. DAMASCELLI, G. FAVA, F. PIZZETTI, U. VERONESI. Cloth DM 48,—; US $ 19.60

38 KOLLER, P. C.: The Role of Chromosomes in Cancer Biology. Cloth DM 48,—; US $ 19.60

39 Current Problems in the Epidemiology of Cancer and Lymphomas. Edited by E. GRUNDMANN and H. TULINIUS (Symposium). Cloth DM 58,—; US $ 23.70

40 LANGLEY, F. A., A. C. CROMPTON: Epithelial Abnormalities of the Cervix Uteri. Cloth DM 58,—; US $ 23.70

41 Tumours in a Tropical Country. A Survey of Uganda (1964—1968). Edited by A. C. TEMPLETON. Cloth DM 72,—; US $ 29.40

42 Breast Cancer: A Challenging Problem. Edited by M. L. GRIEM, E. V. JENSEN, J. E. ULTMANN, and R. W. WISSLER (Symposium). Cloth DM 48,—; US $ 19.60

43 Nomenclature, Methodology and Results of Clinical Trials in Acute Leukemias. Edited by G. MATHÉ, P. POUILLART, and L. SCHWARZENBERG (Symposium). Cloth DM 58,—; US $ 23.70

44 Special Topics in Carcinogenesis. Edited by E. GRUNDMANN (Symposium). Cloth DM 58,—; US $ 23.70

45 KOLDOVSKÝ, P.: Carcinoembryonic Antigens. Cloth DM 38,—; US $ 15.50

46 Diagnosis and Therapy of Malignant Lymphoma. Edited by K. MUSSHOFF (Symposium). Cloth DM 62,—; US $ 25.30

47 Investigation and Stimulation of Immunity in Cancer Patients. Edited by G. MATHÉ and R. WEINER (Symposium). Cloth DM 96,—; US $ 39.20

48 Platinum Coordination Complexes in Cancer Chemotherapy. Edited by T. A. CONNORS and J. J. ROBERTS (Symposium). Cloth DM 68,—; US $ 27.90

49 Complications of Cancer Chemotherapy. Edited by G. MATHÉ and R. K. OLDHAM (Symposium). Cloth DM 58,—; US $ 23.70

50 Cancer Registry. Edited by E. GRUNDMANN and E. PEDERSEN (Symposium). Cloth DM 48,—; US $ 19.70

Special Supplement: Biology of Amphibian Tumors. Edited by M. MIZELL. Cloth DM 96,00; US $ 39.20

In Production

51 Gliomas: Current Concepts in Biology, Diagnosis and Therapy. Edited by J. HEKMATPANAH (Symposium).

Prices are Subject to change without notice